ALSO BY CASEY MEYERS

Aerobic Walking

WALKING

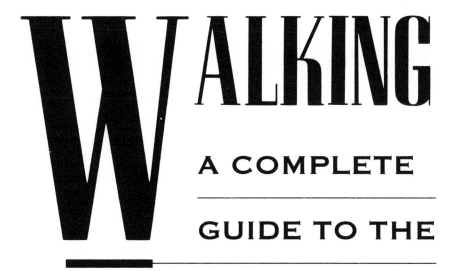

WALKING

A COMPLETE

GUIDE TO THE

COMPLETE

EXERCISE

CASEY MEYERS

RANDOM HOUSE

NEW YORK

All rights reserved under International and Pan-American Copyright Conventions.
Published in the United States by Random House, Inc., New York, and
simultaneously in Canada by Random House of Canada Limited, Toronto.

Library of Congress Cataloging-in-Publication Data
Meyers, Casey.
Walking : a complete guide to the complete exercise / by Casey
Meyers. — 1st ed.
p.   cm.
Includes bibliographical references.
ISBN 0-679-73777-4
1. Walking.   2. Exercise.   I. Title.
GV502.M49   1992

613.7'176—dc20   91-37431

Manufactured in the United States of America
4 6 8 9 7 5
First Edition April 1992

Book design by Debbie Glasserman

The text of this book is set in Stempel Garamond

Illustrations by Pat Stewart

To the three females in my life who have given me so much happiness . . . first, Carol, my staunchest supporter, severest critic, personal confidante, walking companion, devoted wife and eternal love. And then my two loyal "secretaries" who stayed by my desk every minute while I labored writing this book—Goldie, a pretty little blond stray mongrel (mostly cocker spaniel) who happily wandered into my life, and Goulash, my Hungarian Vizsla pointer, who elevates canine love and desire to please to a new level.

Look to your health; and if you have it, praise God, and value it next to a good conscience; for health is the second blessing that we mortals are capable of; a blessing that money cannot buy.

—Izaak Walton

ACKNOWLEDGMENTS

A significant part of the satisfaction of researching and writing this book came from meeting and working with a number of fine people in medicine, exercise, and science who were so very generous in supplying me with their research material, sharing their knowledge, and even critiquing various chapters for me to make sure my manuscript was correct. In that regard, my heartfelt thanks go to Drs. Kenneth Cooper, Boyd Lyles, Neil Gordon, Steven Blair, John Duncan, Howard Palamarchuk, William Byrnes, Jay T. Kearney, and Professors Owen Lovejoy and R. McNeill Alexander. I am extremely grateful also to Dr. George Sheehan for writing the foreword.

Generous help on nutrition came from Kathy Duran and on race walking from Leonard Jansen.

Battling serious illness, my friend and retired English teacher, Virginia Frazier, who gave me guidance on my first book, rose to the occasion again. Connie Heard, working into the wee hours of the morning night after night on her word processor, made sure that I met my manuscript deadline.

Most important, my good friend Dolph Bridgewater and his management team at NaturalSport funded two essential walking studies that put a new spin on walking as an exercise and athletic training aid, without which this book would not have been possible.

And finally, my silent co-author supplied me with key words, phrases, and inspiration during my daily walks. Thank you, God.

FOREWORD

Our beach house on the Jersey Shore overlooks a boardwalk that extends for a mile to the north and five miles to the south. All year long when the weather is right, walkers and runners and cyclists pass by.

The walkers are by far the most numerous. Some are solitary, deep in thought or gazing at the surf and the sea gulls. Others are in groups, couples in quiet conversation, or threesomes talking animatedly. Still others are engaged in earnest effort, arms bent at the elbow and swinging to a rapid cadence. All are experiencing the benefits and the pleasures of walking.

What is happening on our boardwalk is happening all over the country. There has been a renaissance in walking. Walkers are rediscovering what has been known over the centuries. Walking has a global effect on the entire person. It adds hours to one's day and years to one's life. Walking is a superior way to handle stress, and provides the isolation needed for meditation. Not the least of its benefits is the opportunity it gives for creative thinking and solving life's problems.

If these rewards seem similar to the claims made by runners and cyclists and adherents of other activities, it is because they are. Exercise is the generic drug. Walking and running and cycling are simply brands, of which there are many, and all equally effective.

Watching these enthusiasts pass by, I am reminded of the comment Dr. Eliot Joslin, the legendary diabetic specialist, made when asked what the best form of insulin was. "All insulins are good insulins if you know how to use them." This is certainly true about exercise. All exercises are good exercises if you know how to use them. And of all these exercises, walking has the longest history, the best pedigree, the most distinguished practitioners. Walking was Nature's first exercise, and has been recommended by authorities over the centuries.

In the first book totally devoted to exercise, published in 1555, Christobol Mendez writes: "The best and most beneficial exercise is walking." Mendez gives many reasons for selecting walking. It fulfills all the requirements and is so easy that no matter where you are you can do it. Even more important, according to Mendez, walking offers many pleasures and joys. He points out that you can observe, read, converse, sing, meditate and practice all your mental skills like imagination, cogitation, and memory.

Harry Andrews, the most highly respected track coach at the turn of the century, was another proponent of walking. Andrews included among his athletes Walter George, the world's best at the mile, and the incomparable Alfie Shrubb, who once held all the world's records for distances from two miles to fifteen miles, and many others runners, boxers and cyclists of the time.

Andrews regarded walking as fundamental to all training. "Experience tells me," he writes, "that walking should represent the groundwork for any system of training." It did not matter to him what sport you were in, whether running, boxing, fencing, cycling or rowing; walking as a primary exercise was applicable to all. According to Andrews, "It gave by far the greatest benefit of any form of training in its result."

For those interested only in fitness, walking was his recommended activity. He saw no need to do anything else. It was a superior way to reduce weight and there was no need to worry about pace. "The best advice I can give," he wrote, "is to make your own pace—the pace, in fact, that will suit you best. This pace will almost certainly be an average of four miles an hour."

In the lines above I have presented evidence from the distant past. In this book Casey Meyers brings us up to date on research, both his own and that of others, proving that walking is for everybody. The overweight, out-of-shape beginner, the accomplished athlete, and everyone in between will benefit by making walking part of their lives.

—George Sheehan, M.D.
December 1991

PREFACE

Without any promotion or publicity by a celebrity, sports hero, or athletic shoe company, with no fanfare of any kind, the exercise-walking movement quietly launched itself in the mid-1980s. At first it was just a spontaneous trickle of people—mostly women —taking to the sidewalks, parks, and shopping malls to do something that felt natural, physically rewarding, and mentally stimulating and that was noninjurious. The more walking they did, the more they realized that this was the exercise they were all meant to do.

From this quiet beginning, the word spread and exercise walking gathered momentum, propelled along by a ground swell of common sense. People who had dropped out of other exercises or abandoned exercise equipment because of injury or boredom joined in and found that exercise walking is safe, effective, and enjoyable. Whereas walking made sense to the average person, most of the exercise experts were still promoting running, high-impact aerobics, cycling, swimming, rope jumping, and use of a variety of exercise equipment, such as rowing machines and exercise cycles. In a nation obsessed with youth, speed, glitz, and glamour, walking was too plain and ordinary. It was the ugly duckling of exercise.

Even though exercise walking is now the number-one exercise in the United States and growing each year, it is still not given the status it deserves by many exercise professionals. For athletic conditioning, it is universally rejected by coaches and athletes because they do not know that the walking gait can produce more comprehensive exercise results than any other exercise or exercise equipment. Contrary to popular belief, walking can produce injury-free aerobic capacities and/or cross-training results not attainable by running. I am convinced exercise walking should be the foundation exercise in every physical-fitness regimen, and you will be too when you find out how versatile it is.

Understanding the origin of bipedality and how our locomotion system evolved makes it easier to understand the biomechanics of the walking gait. As bipeds, we have two gaits of locomotion— walking and running. How they differ as *gaits* determines how each functions as an exercise or sport. Recent walking studies that I have been associated with at the Institute for Aerobics Research and the United States Olympic Training Center have demonstrated that walking has far more exercise potential than we have been led to believe and far more than we are utilizing.

Describing the human anatomy and how our locomotion system functions requires the use of anatomical and biomechanical terms not familiar to most people. I confess many were not familiar to me. I'll try to make this book not only informative but easy to read. When it is necessary to use scientific words that are not part of the average person's vocabulary, I will insert their definitions at the point of usage so that you will not have to scramble for a dictionary.

For example, a word in the foregoing paragraph that will be used extensively through the book is *biomechanical*. That may not be a word that is readily understood by all. The *Random House Dictionary of the English Language*, unabridged, which is my reference source, defines *biomechanics* as "the study of the action of external and internal forces on the living body, especially on the skeletal system." Essentially *biomechanics* describes how our arms and legs function as we move about.

I have researched the antiquity of the walking gait from an evolutionist's point of view, and evolution is occasionally referred to through the book. Many Christians accept the theory of evolution; however, Christian creationists believe that the walking gait came into being 6,000 years ago in the Garden of Eden when God created Adam and Eve. I respect all religious beliefs and ask those who are uneasy with the concept of evolution to insert mentally the origin and time frame of creation they believe in when the word is mentioned.

Whether the walking gait evolved over millions of years or was specifically designed by God and put into place 6,000 years ago does not alter the fact that, although we may worship differently, biomechanically we *all* walk the same today. Unfortunately, most people do not walk enough. In the highly mechanized Western industrialized countries, walking as a form of locomotion has been reduced to a minor role. The abnormal reduction of this fundamental human physical activity has led to obesity and a wide range of health-related problems for a large segment of the population. For the extremely sedentary, it has even led to a reduced life span. That's the downside. The upside is that most of this can be reversed with increased walking, which more than any other exercise will contribute to the health of your body, mind, and spirit.

I truly hope the information and research I have assembled in this book will inspire you to become an exercise walker. Join me and the millions of others who have already discovered that a happier, healthier life is just a walk away.

CONTENTS

WALKING

1

EXERCISE:
THE OUNCE
OF PREVENTION

The late Redd Foxx, star of the old TV show *Sanford and Son* and a new one called *The Royal Family*, was a comedian known for his irreverent brand of humor. In one of his TV appearances, Foxx said the reason he was against exercise was "Someday all of those health and fitness nuts are gonna be lyin' in the hospital dyin' of *nuthin*!" Given the alternatives, "nuthin" isn't a bad way to go. As implausible as Foxx's comment seems, there's probably a grain of truth in it. Ironically, Foxx died suddenly of a heart attack at the age of 68 while rehearsing an episode of his new show.

Compelling evidence reveals that regular physical activity is beneficial for cardiovascular health, weight control, and reduction of symptoms of depression, depressed mood, and anxiety. In a nation where it is estimated that 50 million men and 60 million women between the ages of 18 and 79 are "too fat," the weight-control problem opens up a large set of other health-related diseases. Excessive fat contributes to an increased risk of hypertension, adult diabetes, gallbladder disease, degenerative joint disease and gout, some types of cancer, and impairment of cardiac function resulting from the increased work load on the heart.

The foregoing clearly indicates that physical activity and exercise are directly related to improved health. People who remain sedentary certainly don't have to worry about dying of "nuthin." In fact, being sedentary is now a known contributing factor to a shortened life expectancy. It may seem unbelievable, but, given the choice between being physically active for a better quality of life and the possibility of living longer and remaining sedentary, the vast majority of the population has opted for the latter.

The eighties was considered the health and fitness decade. Fitness clubs, aerobics classes, marathons, athletic shoes, athletic clothes, and Jane Fonda's "Go for the burn" were all the rage. While a few people became motivated exercisers, the actual numbers reveal that there was more conversation about exercise than commitment to it. Most people bought jogging outfits because they were comfortable to wear while watching television. They never worked up a sweat.

Less than 10 percent of the population exercises three or more times a week at a level vigorous enough to improve cardiorespiratory fitness, according to the U.S. Department of Health and Human Services. In its 692-page book *Healthy People 2000: National Health Promotion and Disease Prevention Objectives*, published in 1990, the department assesses the current status of the nation's health and lays out objectives for the nineties.

Heart disease continues to be the number-one cause of death in the United States, according to the department. If less than 10 percent of the population is exercising enough to improve cardiorespiratory fitness, what is the other 90 percent doing? As you might expect, not much. The department reports that "25 percent of adults report *no* leisure-time physical activity and the prevalence of sedentary behavior increases with advancing age." This is a worrisome statistic because, by the year 2000, people over 65 will be 13 percent of the population, and during this decade the most rapid population increase will be among those over 85 years of age.

Nationally, only 22 percent of adults engage in at least 30 minutes of light to moderate physical activity five or more times a week. Believe it or not, this group may be better off than the few who brag about running a marathon. As we look back with regret at the many excesses of the eighties, we can include several exercise doctrines, such as no pain, no gain; you can never do too much exercise; and marathon running creates an invulnerability to heart attacks. We now know better.

FATHER OF AEROBICS
PREACHES MODERATION

"I've heard that while exercise will make you physically fit, it doesn't actually contribute to your health—is that true?" With the energy and speed of a quarter horse breaking from a starting gate, Dr. Kenneth Cooper was out of his chair and in front of the projection screen. He motioned for the projectionist to put up the slide that he had given him before the program started, in anticipation of a question just like this. If a shill had been placed in the audience, the question could not have been phrased better to suit Dr. Cooper.

It came from a magazine editor who, with other members of the press, had come to hear the details of a major study on exercise walking that had been conducted at the Institute for Aerobics Research in Dallas. It was April 11, 1991, and I had flown to New York City to be part of the program with Dr. Cooper (the founder and head of the institute) and Dr. John Duncan (the researcher who conducted the study). My role was to explain the walking technique I taught the study participants.

Dr. Kenneth Cooper is best known as "the father of aerobics." He wrote the book *Aerobics* in 1968, and the word *aerobic* has since passed into our language. In 1986, the *Oxford English Dictionary* asked Dr. Cooper to write the definition of the word he'd coined for the dictionary's new edition. He defined it as "a method of physical exercise for producing beneficial changes in the respiratory and circulatory systems by activities which require only a modest increase in oxygen intake and so can be maintained."

Dr. Cooper presides over a 30-acre complex in north Dallas that he started in 1970. It includes the Institute for Aerobics Research, the internationally renowned Cooper Clinic, the Cooper Wellness Program, and a 3,000-member Aerobics Activity Center. A prolific writer of health and fitness books, Dr. Cooper is also a sought-after speaker. With missionary-like zeal, he travels extensively, preaching the benefits of exercise and preventive medicine to corporations and health organizations.

That morning we had breakfast together and talked about the importance of exercise and physical activity as they relate to each individual's health and the health of the nation. Dr. Cooper told me then what he was now anxious to tell the assembled press: "We

must get the word out to everyone that moderate exercise, something as simple as walking 30 to 45 minutes a day at a brisk pace,
will produce the moderate fitness level which is associated with a
greatly reduced risk of death."

Dr. Cooper also reminisced about how much more the exercise
community knows, and how much more *he* knows, now than 20
years ago or even 10 years ago. He said, "You know, Casey, I
was wrong when I wrote *Aerobics* in 1968. I believed more exercise
was better, that you could not run a good thing into the ground.
Now I strongly advocate moderation." Then the man who, along
with Jim Fixx (a friend of his), had gotten the nation running and
jogging said something that was music to my ears: "I think people
should walk more and run less."

When the charts flashed on the screen, I knew what was coming.
Dr. Cooper has a commanding voice and staccato-like delivery
that a tent-and-sawdust traveling evangelist would break a couple
of commandments for. He soon had everyone riveted as he described the importance of the charts (see Figure 1.1). The main
thrust of his message was simple: "If more people moved from
sedentary living to a moderate level of fitness, the result would be
a major impact on death rates."

The charts were constructed from data compiled in a landmark
study conducted by the Institute for Aerobics Research that involved 10,224 men and 3,120 women over more than eight years
and was the first scientific study of this magnitude to prove a direct
relationship between physical fitness and increased life expectancy
(as much as two to three years). Equally important, the fitness
level required to produce the most significant results is well within
the range of the general population—that is, people like you and
me. The elitism of marathon running contributed little extra from
a longevity standpoint. On a risk-reward basis for an average exerciser, marathons are obsolete.

Dr. Cooper stressed that "moderate fitness" differed by only a
few percentage points from high fitness. It is interesting to note
that highly fit women did not fare as well as the "moderate" group.
Dr. Cooper concluded, "This study and other recent research suggest that sedentary living habits and low levels of physical fitness
are very important risk factors for early death and deserve increased
attention by the public and the medical profession."

1984: A PIVOTAL YEAR IN EXERCISE

In July 1984, Jim Fixx, the author of *The Complete Book of Running*, died of a heart attack while running on a country road in New England. His book, published seven years earlier, had launched the nation on a jogging, running, and marathon binge. Fixx's name had become synonymous with the running movement, and his death was chilling news to even the most ardent runner.

Confusion and controversy about running and exercise—much of it created by Fixx himself—arose out of his untimely death. In *Second Book of Running*, Fixx wrote, "Heart attacks, while not unknown in trained runners, are so rare as to be of negligible probability." Then he quoted approvingly a doctor who declared, "The only thing that can kill a healthy runner, other than cars and buses, is heat stroke." Ironically, Fixx's death disproved those unwarranted claims, and the running movement has never regained its national allure.

The proponents of exercise were scrambling for explanations of Fixx's death and were in general disarray when, in the fall of 1984, *The Exercise Myth* by Dr. Henry A. Solomon hit the bookstores. It said just what fat, sedentary people wanted to hear. Don't do any vigorous exercise because you might drop dead. Dr. Solomon fired a vitriolic salvo directly at the exercise proponents. He aimed his initial shot at his fellow doctors: "The medical professional provides a legitimacy for exercise where otherwise there would be none." This statement ultimately proved as extreme and wrong as some of those made by Fixx.

As a practicing New York City cardiologist and a member of the faculty at Cornell University Medical College, Dr. Solomon, who could not be written off as a quack, seemed to relish his attack on exercise. He sought to discredit it thoroughly. The last two sentences of his book were "The exercise fad is a folly and a danger. It only takes you to spread the word." Between the first chapter and these closing sentences, Solomon ridiculed stress tests, vigorous exercise, and most participants, as well as doctors, involved with exercise.

Fortunately, between Fixx's death and the appearance of Solomon's groundless book, cooler heads were sorting out the facts about exercise. In September 1984, at the U.S. government's prestigious Centers for Disease Control in Atlanta, a blue-ribbon panel of physicians and exercise physiologists met in what was called the

Workshop on Epidemiologic and Public Health Aspects of Physical Activity and Exercise. That's a mouthful, so I will herein refer to it simply as the CDC Workshop. *Epidemiology* is also a word you won't hear at the average lunch counter, and the dictionary defines it as "the branch of medicine dealing with the incidence and prevalence of disease in large populations and with detection of the source and cause of epidemics of infectious disease."

Papers on various aspects of physical activity and exercise were presented and discussed. A paper presented by Dr. William Haskell of Stanford, Dr. Henry Montoye of the University of Wisconsin, Madison, and Dr. Diane Orenstein of the CDC stated: "Physical activity that appears to provide the most diverse health benefits consists of dynamic, rhythmic contractions of large muscles that transport the body over distance or against gravity at a moderate intensity relative to capacity for extended periods of time during which 200 to 400 kilocalories [calories to us] are expended." The authors added, "For optimal health benefits, such activity should be performed daily or at least every other day." Read that again, because it sure sounds to me like a roundabout way of saying we should all take a good long walk.

Even in 1984 there was ample evidence that moderate exercise has a positive effect on health. Drs. Haskell, Montoye, and Orenstein pointed out: "The greatest benefits are achieved when the least active individuals become moderately active; much less benefit is apparent when the already active individual becomes extremely active." Figure 1.1 clearly confirms this. It can be said that marathons contribute more to the runners' cocktail party conversation than to their health.

There is considerable confusion for many people about the difference between physical activity and exercise. The CDC Workshop defined *physical activity* as "any bodily movement produced by skeletal muscles that results in energy expenditure"; and *exercise* as "planned, structured, and repetitive bodily movement done to improve or maintain one or more components of *physical fitness*." Those last two words are also defined. *Physical fitness* is "a set of attributes that people have or achieve that relates to the ability to perform physical activity." And *those* last two words, *physical activity*, bring us back to where we started. Washing the windows or raking leaves is physical activity. Walking 3 miles every morning before you go to work is structured exercise. Being able to do either without undue fatigue is a measure of physical fitness.

FIGURE 1.1A

Physical fitness and risk of all-cause mortality in men

AGE-ADJUSTED DEATH RATE / 10,000

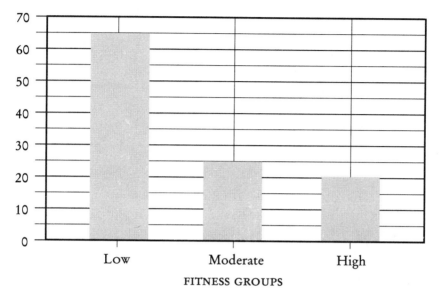

FITNESS GROUPS

FIGURE 1.1B

Physical fitness and risk of all-cause mortality in women

AGE-ADJUSTED DEATH RATE / 10,000

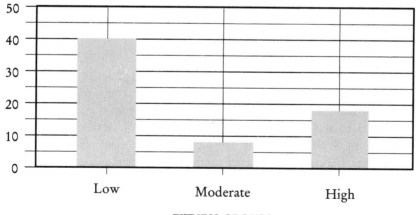

FITNESS GROUPS

SOURCE: S.N. Blair et al., "Physical fitness and all-cause mortality," *JAMA* 262(17): 2395–2401, 1989.

It is important to distinguish between health and fitness when contemplating exercise. It is possible to be highly fit but unhealthy, as Jim Fixx was. For health and longevity, you need only walk regularly at a brisk pace, as the Institute for Aerobics Research study suggests. For a high level of aerobic fitness, you will have to exercise at an elevated level of intensity, as described in Chapter 6. Aerobic fitness contributes to your quality of life *and* longevity by giving you the physical capacity to ski, play tennis, play racquetball, or undertake any other activity requiring a high energy level. Simply stated, *moderate exercise contributes to your health, whereas high-intensity exercise contributes to your health and fitness.*

As in all things in life, you cannot take out of exercise more than you put in. In my personal walking program, I have found that high-intensity exercise walking has a residual "feel-good" effect. The harder I walk, the better I feel. That will not necessarily be true for everyone, however, so the primary consideration for your exercise-walking program should be *consistency*, irrespective of intensity.

The broad conclusions of the CDC Workshop embraced exercise and increased physical activity wholeheartedly. The benefits of exercise are not a myth. When done consistently, exercise contributes to a wide range of health benefits, including quality and quantity of life. Exercise is also deemed indispensable as an aid to weight control. The fact that you are reading this book may indicate your good intention to exercise. The numbers who follow through with a lifetime exercise program, however, are very small, and, according to the CDC Workshop, "The reasons why people do or do not exercise are largely unknown."

There have always been a few enlightened, dedicated walkers, but it was in 1984 that the exercise-walking movement quietly started to attract big numbers. Between the fear created by Jim Fixx's death and the mindless confusion sown by Henry Solomon's book, people, without any urging from the exercise experts, decided that walking was a safe exercise compromise. As late as 1984, however, very little research had been done on or attention paid to walking by the exercise community. The CDC Workshop observed, "Empirical data about the risk of walking, the most common activity, are absent." Clearly the people who had already become exercise walkers were ahead of the professionals.

EXERCISE AND THE MEDICAL GAP

Somewhere in the front of every exercise book is a warning to consult your doctor before exercising. I will insert my own warning right here, with emphasis: *Do not do any exercise recommended in this book until you have permission from your doctor*. These caveats, however, are probably more for the protection of the author and publisher than for the exerciser, because, except for patients who are in obvious life-threatening situations, most doctors are ill-equipped to advise about exercise.

In the October 1988 issue of *The Physician and Sportsmedicine*, a study titled "Exercise Medicine in Medical Education in the United States" reviewed 92 U.S. medical school bulletins, which showed that only 4 schools offer exercise medicine as part of *required* undergraduate course work. Thirty-one schools offer exercise information on an *elective* basis, but 57 schools offer *no* formal exercise instruction. Thus, the vast majority of medical students in the United States do not receive any formal instruction on the medical aspects of exercise during their four-year undergraduate education. According to the study's authors, the situation has not changed significantly since 1975, when a similar study was done. This is why I said the warning to consult your physician before exercise may be more for the writer's protection than the exerciser's.

Most practicing physicians have insufficient knowledge and training to prescribe an appropriate exercise regimen. This is a sad state of affairs, because many people who exercise or who plan to start exercising expect their physicians, as their primary health-care providers, to answer their questions about exercise. The study just cited reported: "The most frequently asked questions relate to health benefits and to specific prescriptions (frequency, duration, intensity, and mode)."

The lead article in the June 1988 issue of *The Physician and Sportsmedicine* was titled "Sports Medicine: Where Do We Go from Here." Dr. Kenneth E. Powell, chief of the Behavior Epidemiology and Evaluation Branch of the CDC, said that, for the most part, "the medical community has been reluctant to accept and act upon the scientific evidence that regular physical exercise has beneficial health effects." He also pointed out: "The medical community seems to passively accept that regular physical activity is good for people, yet in practice they seldom prescribe it to their patients."

The therapeutic effects of exercise as a form of preventive medicine are well established, and I have attempted to assemble in this book all the information you need to proceed with a safe, effective, noninjurious exercise program. In addition to extensive research, I have had the medical advice and counsel of Dr. Boyd Lyles, one of the top preventive-medicine clinicians at the Cooper Clinic. Further guidance was provided by Dr. Neil Gordon, a medical doctor as well as director of exercise physiology at the Institute for Aerobics Research, who supplied me with the latest research information and exercise prescriptions for a variety of illnesses.

If your doctor advises you to exercise and prescribes specific exercises in terms of frequency, duration, and intensity, by all means follow his or her advice. The information in this book is not intended in any way to usurp your doctor's instructions to you. If for any reason my advice conflicts with your doctor's, *always* follow your doctor's recommendations. New procedures, new medications, and a variety of extenuating circumstances could alter the desired effects of an exercise program. Whether the information comes from this book or from your doctor, the most important consideration is that you be on a lifetime exercise program.

FIX IT BEFORE IT'S BROKEN

There's a popular saying, "If it ain't broke, don't fix it." Although that may be sound advice for many things in life, when it comes to health, it could be deadly advice. By the time someone's health is "broke," it may be too late to fix it. The cumulative effects of an unhealthy life-style sometimes cannot be undone. The time to fix your health with exercise and proper nutrition is before it's broken.

In *Healthy People 2000*, the Department of Health and Human Services lists the national goals for "health promotion." Of the eight categories that affect the nation's health, they list "physical activity and fitness" as number one and "nutrition" next. In this sedentary, underexercised nation, millions of people consume too much dietary fat and are literally sitting and eating themselves into a diseased state and early death. There is no longer any disagreement in the medical profession about this fact. The only question is, Are you one of those people?

Although a case can be made that medical schools and doctors are lagging behind in training and counseling on exercise, an even greater case can be made that people would prefer to take a "magic pill" than to break out of their sedentary rut. Dr. Boyd Lyles confirms that even when exercise would be more effective and beneficial over the long term than prescription drugs, most people prefer drugs.

Statistics reveal that the majority of the general population is reluctant to exercise, and most doctors do not believe they can alter their patients' attitude about exercise. The CDC Workshop cited a study published in the *New England Journal of Medicine* that found that less than 10 percent of physicians believed they were successful in helping patients change their behaviors. There is no magic pill to cure lethargy; you must be willing to make a few life-style changes for your health's sake.

In one of our many meetings while I was researching this book, Dr. Lyles said to me, "It is hard to believe, but 65 percent of all deaths are life-style-related." Although this book is about exercise, with one chapter devoted to nutrition, I would be remiss if I did not point out that the most damaging of all life-style activities is *smoking*. You can't walk enough miles or eat enough low-fat foods to undo the damage caused to the body by smoking. As Dr. Lyles put it, "Nothing even comes close to smoking as the biggest cause of preventable death. Smoking is in a class by itself because it is a major contributor to premature death from heart disease, stroke, lung cancer, and emphysema. There's nothing people can do to themselves that will kill them over a broader spectrum of diseases than smoking."

Right behind smoking is being sedentary and consuming a high-fat diet. This combination generally leads to being overweight, which brings on other health problems. Dr. Lyles said that the two are so interrelated that they can hardly be separated. Both are major contributors to the prevalence of heart disease. Throw in the high incidence of alcohol and drug abuse, and it is a rare individual in this country who dies of natural causes—or, as Redd Foxx said, of "nuthin." The majority are literally poisoning themselves to death.

Having given you all the grim reasons you should make the commitment to a healthy life-style and start exercising, let me give you the real reason regular exercisers continue to exercise: *it makes them feel better physically and mentally.*

I remember a conversation I had with Dr. Kenneth Cooper. He said, "Casey, even though we can prove that exercise can prolong life two or three years, I am not convinced that this will motivate people to exercise. Ninety-five percent of the people I know who exercise regularly do so because it makes them feel better, pure and simple." If I can make a lifetime exercise walker out of you, it *may* help you to live longer, but I *guarantee* it will make you feel better physically and give you a happier, more positive outlook on life.

This is just the first chapter; there are fourteen more ahead of you, so, before you read the message, maybe you should know a little bit about the messenger. I am a retired businessman. I have a fairly comfortable retirement income and a compelling desire to live a long, healthy life. For good reasons: I have a beautiful wife, whom I adore, two fine grown children, two crackerjack grandsons, an old, grumpy cocker spaniel who is the queen of our house, and a Vizsla quail dog whom I love like another child. These are my worldly riches, and I want to enjoy them for as long as possible. Quantity *and* quality of life are important to me.

I was 50 years old before I made my first attempt at exercising. I finally made it stick on the third try, when I was 52, but I don't really know why: I just stayed with it. Over the years my weight had ballooned by 52 pounds and four suit sizes. I was a hard-driving businessman more interested in my bottom line than in my waistline. Exercise was the last thing I wanted to waste time on. Believe me, even today I am not an exercise nut, and I will not try to turn you into one.

When this book is published, I will be 64 years old. On my last treadmill fitness test, conducted by Dr. Lyles at the Cooper Clinic during my annual physical, I rated "superior" (the highest rating) for a 50-year-old and "excellent" (second-highest rating) for *30 years old and younger.* Physically I am in better shape than when I was 30. I am 6 feet, 2 inches tall and weigh 182, with body fat of 16 percent. My weight hasn't fluctuated 2 pounds in eight years, and the only exercise I do is walk. If you are looking for the mythical fountain of youth, I promise you that exercise walking will get you closer to it than anything else you can do. It will help you stall the aging process.

In this book, I promise to give you the road map to a healthier, happier life, but it will require some modest behavioral commitments. Unlike other exercises you may have tried, exercise walking will not bore you or injure you. It can't be done in a La-Z-Boy recliner in front of the TV, however. You'll have to get up off your rusty, dusty rear end and start moving.

With walking, I will show you how to take charge of your life mentally and physically in a way you never thought possible. You will exercise in a pleasing, natural way. I caution you not to become impatient with walking; it works its magic gradually. Walking will take your unfit body and troubled mind and gently massage them into a state of readiness to battle life's problems or to enjoy more of life's pleasures.

I was lucky when I finally became an exerciser. I was sedentary, overweight, and unfit but had not yet paid a health price for it. Don't put off your walking program another day; the time to exercise is *before* you have health problems. Starting to exercise while you are still healthy is like following the old Chinese proverb "A wise man does not wait until he is thirsty to dig a well."

It is quite a stretch from Redd Foxx to a Chinese proverb, but I hope I have been able to arouse your interest in walking for exercise. It truly is the ounce of prevention that's worth a pound of cure. The walking gait has been fundamental to human life for longer than most people realize.

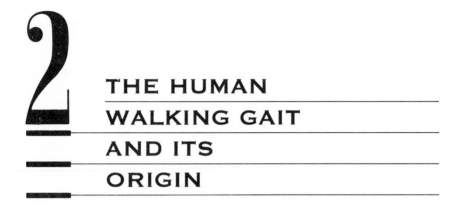

2

THE HUMAN
WALKING GAIT
AND ITS
ORIGIN

The Pufferbelly restaurant is in an old railroad station about a mile from the Kent State University campus. Sitting at a corner table with me, anthropologist Dr. Owen Lovejoy pensively poked at his salad with his fork, then looked up and said, "If I could get my hands on a 6-million-year-old pelvis, it would tell me a lot." I had just asked Dr. Lovejoy what kind of anthropological find he would need to determine when bipedality and the human walking gait were in their earliest stages. During my research for this book, I had read his treatise "Evolution of Human Walking," which appeared in the November 1988 issue of *Scientific American*.

In his article, Dr. Lovejoy explored the origin of bipedal walking, its biomechanics, and its pluses and minuses. I traveled to Kent, Ohio, to discuss this and one of his other anthropological accomplishments. Dr. Lovejoy had helped to reconstruct and analyze the important 3-million-year-old female hominid skeleton that was discovered in northern Ethiopia in 1974. It was this skeleton that established our present knowledge of the antiquity of bipedal walking.

LUCY AND THE EVOLUTION OF
HUMAN WALKING

In the preface, I said I would give the definitions as we went along for terms you might not be familiar with. Right out of the chute we hit the word *hominid*, which is not commonly used at the average American breakfast table. I didn't know what it meant either, so I looked it up for both of us. My dictionary defines it this way: "any of the modern or extinct bipedal primates of the family Hominidae, including all species of the genera Homo and Australopithecus." This female skeleton is the extinct *Australopithecus* (pronounced ah stra lo pith´ e kas), the oldest known genus of Hominidae. We are the *Homo sapiens* species (modern man), and about 3 to 4 million years of evolution separate us from *Australopithecus*.

The anthropologists who made the discovery officially labeled the skeleton A.L. 288-1 but affectionately called her Lucy, a name taken from the Beatles' song "Lucy in the Sky with Diamonds," popular in the expedition's camp at that time. Lucy was a small adult female, 3 feet, 8 inches tall and weighing about 65 pounds. What is most significant is that Lucy's skeleton reveals that she was as adept at upright walking as we are. It proves conclusively that bipedality was fully in place 3 million years ago. Bipedal walking became the primary gait of locomotion for all of the species that followed Lucy and ultimately for us humans.

Dr. Lovejoy told me that our walking gait is about 98 percent identical with Lucy's and that the differences are "just a few biomechanical subtleties. The most obvious morphological [structural] difference between Lucy and modern man appears to be the result of different degrees of encephalization [brain development]," he said. Lucy had a head and brain about the size of a chimpanzee's.

We humans, by contrast, developed a much bigger brain and got smarter—in some ways, maybe too smart for our own good. Lucy could walk, but she couldn't talk. She did not have the ability to form articulate words, so there was as yet no language. She had to forage for her food every day; there was no agriculture. The earliest recognizable stone tools are about 2 million years old, so Lucy was even a million years too early for the Stone Age. "It was only 2 million years from the first primitive stone tools to the industrial revolution about 150 years ago," Dr. Lovejoy pointed out to me. "In the last 100,000 years, we went from Neanderthal to Cro-Magnon—modern man. Agriculture and domesticated animals came on the scene about 10,000 years ago; language, cultures, and religions appeared, and the wheel was invented. In terms of time from a geological reference, all of this occurred quicker than you can blink your eye."

The encephalization process yielded new locomotion systems as well, ones that have rendered our 3-million-year-old walking gait nearly obsolete. In the last 100 years, the walking gait has come to be viewed by most people in Western industrialized countries as the locomotion system of last resort. Trains, planes, and automobiles have become our choices for traveling great distances. For moving shorter distances, motorcycles, golf carts, riding mowers, farm tractors, escalators, elevators, and moving walkways—a real oxymoron—are a few of our other choices.

We have created a variety of mechanical locomotion systems that require little or no physical effort. Have we gotten too smart, perhaps? For instance, by riding more and walking less, are we shortchanging the physical-activity requirements for a longer, healthier life?

In a Harvard School of Public Health study on the connection between exercise and weight gain, the authors stated: "In his hundreds of thousands of years of evolution, man did not have any opportunity for sedentary life except very recently. An inactive life for man is as recent (and as 'abnormal') a development as caging is for an animal. In this light, it is not surprising that some of the usual adjustment mechanisms would prove inadequate."

Over the past few years, millions of people have rediscovered walking as a source of physical activity and regular exercise. Some doctors and exercise physiologists offer words of caution, however, and speculate on possible injury. Can it be possible that, after at least 3 million years of usage, the oldest form of locomotion is flawed? Or has walking been relegated to such a lesser role in our lives that we have forgotten that at one time it was the only way the human species and all our extinct ancestors could move about?

An early example of injury concern was voiced at the CDC Workshop I referred to in the previous chapter. In the section "The Risks of Exercise: A Public Health View of Injuries and Hazards," the three reporting physicians postulated: "unknown are the injuries and hazards associated with walking and the rates at which they occur. *We hypothesize that walkers share similar risks with runners"* (my emphasis). Fortunately, in the 8 years since that hypothesis, we have found that there are *no* similarities between the risk of a running injury and that of a walking injury. Later in this chapter and in the next, you will find out why.

A director of the Center for Locomotion Studies at a major East Coast college was quoted in the April–May 1988 issue of *The Walking Magazine* as saying: "There's a great deal of interest now in studying walking, as it gains popularity as an exercise form. *And, of course, there will be even more interest as we start seeing more walking-related injuries in the future"* (my emphasis). It is now four years later. Where are all those "walking-related injuries"?

In fairness to these two sources, I must say that they, like many others, view walking as an "exercise" instead of as the primary gait of locomotion for humans. Think about this: whether biped (two-legged) or quadruped (four-legged), there aren't any examples in the scientific literature of animals incurring injury—other than accidental—when functioning in their primary gait.

Biological necessity is the sine qua non of evolution. The walking gait is fundamental to the survivability of all terrestrial species. We are designed to walk and walk and walk. It was the speculations and unfounded concerns about walking's injury potential that prompted me to seek out Dr. Lovejoy. I was starting from square one, but I had a gut feeling that a complete understanding of the origin, longevity, and biomechanics of the walking gait would clear up any confusion about its effectiveness and limitations as an exercise.

Dr. Lovejoy had generously set side his late afternoon and evening to explain all this to me. He also patiently helped me translate the esoteric language of human anatomy and its biomechanics into the everyday language of people like you and me. It was a fascinating discussion.

"One of the most distinctive features of the human species is our upright mode of locomotion, which is found only in human beings and our immediate ancestors," Dr. Lovejoy pointed out. All other primates are basically quadrupedal, and with good reason. "Walking on two limbs instead of four has many drawbacks. It deprives us of speed and agility and all but eliminates our capacity to climb trees, which yield many important primate foods, such as fruits and nuts."

I was curious. "Why would a 6-million-year-old pelvis be helpful in establishing walking's earliest development?" I asked.

"The distinctive pelvic features of a biped reflect the very different mechanics of two- and four-legged locomotion," Dr. Lovejoy responded. "In order to propel itself, any terrestrial mammal—human, horse, or dog, for example—must apply a force against the ground in a direction opposite to the direction of travel."

Walking works this way. If you want to go north, your back foot pushes against the ground in a southerly direction. A horse goes east when its alternating back hooves push against the ground in a westerly direction. The role of the pelvis becomes critical to bipedal and quadrupedal locomotion because the pelvis is the key anchor point for the bones and muscles involved in the propulsion systems.

"A quadruped has a greater amount of horizontal forward thrust than a biped; that's why we lost speed and agility when we became upright," Dr. Lovejoy explained. "In the quadrupedal posture, the center of mass lies well forward of the hind limbs. Our upright posture, in contrast, places our center of mass almost directly over the foot. We lose horizontal thrust and thus lose speed." Here's another uncommon term—*center of mass*—which the dictionary defines as "the point at which the entire mass of a body may be considered concentrated for some purposes." It is like a point on the body where, if you stuck a rod through it, it would be evenly balanced in all directions, just as a wheel is around its axle.

One only has to look at Figure 2.1 to see what Dr. Lovejoy means by *center of mass*. The horse in Figure 2.1A has two circles on the front part of its body. The small black circle within the big circle around the chest, neck, head, and shoulders is its hypothetical center of mass. The overlapping circle, at the back, is around the large muscles and pelvis, commonly known as the hindquarters. That propulsion area is where the horse and other quadrupeds generate their great forward horizontal thrust and speed.

Conversely, the circles on the human in Figure 2.1B are literally stacked on top of one another. The big top circle is around the rib cage and upper body, generally called the torso or trunk. The small black circle within that is the hypothetical human center of mass. The overlapping bottom circle is around our propulsion system—the buttocks, pelvis, and legs. With this biomechanical arrangement, horizontal forward thrust is minimal. It is obvious that we aren't built for running speed.

You can easily demonstrate for yourself how we lack the forward thrust of a quadruped. Simply stand with your pelvis directly under your trunk, as in Figure 2.1B. With your legs together and straight at the knee, push against the ground with your forefoot. Notice that your ankles rotate as you push and that you don't go forward: you simply rise vertically, ending up on your toes like a ballet dancer.

How do we engage our walking gait, then, so we can move forward instead of vertically? Dr. Lovejoy explained it this way: "In order to propel our upright trunk, we must reposition our center of mass ahead of one leg. The trailing limb, which includes the foot, is lengthened to produce a ground reaction—the foot pushing off—while the other leg is swung forward to keep the trunk from falling."

The walking gait is actually a sequential lifting and falling of the body as our weight-bearing leg passes under us and becomes the trailing leg. The foot of that leg pushes against the ground, and our trunk (or center of mass), is thrust up and forward. Then it begins to fall. The lead leg swinging forward stops its fall as the heel is planted in front. This then becomes the weight-bearing leg as the body passes over it and the process called the human walking gait repeats itself. That's how we walk. We do it every day—we just don't do enough of it.

It is the combination of our unusual locomotion system and the development of our massive brain that makes us unique in the animal kingdom. Our locomotion system dictates what we can do long term for physical exercise, and I believe our advanced brain development dictates what we will do. We are too smart to do unnatural, boring physical exercise for long periods.

THE BIOMECHANICS OF WALKING

In the five years since my first book, *Aerobic Walking*, was published, I have worked with thousands of people in walking clinics coast to coast. During this time two things have struck me as funny. First, everybody *drove* to the clinic to learn how to walk, and, second, almost all knew more about how their cars functioned than about how their bodies did.

FIGURE 2.1A

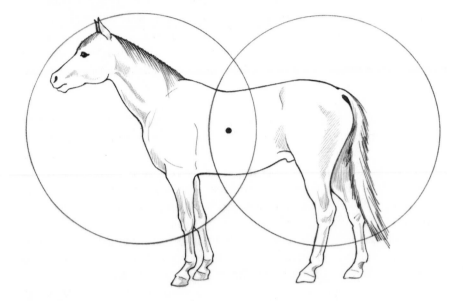

FIGURE 2.1B

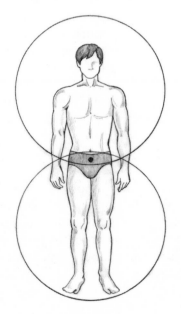

I believe I know why. Human physiology and medical terms are intimidating. Practically everything is in Latin—which is Greek to me. The body isn't much more complicated than an automobile, however, when it comes to knowing a few of the basic parts and how they function. If you can understand a mechanical locomotion system, you can understand a biomechanical one. Certainly, if I can understand it, anybody can.

It is essential for you to know how the human musculoskeletal system (muscles and skeleton) is put together and how it functions biomechanically in the walking and running gaits. I guarantee that this will make it easier for you to understand why and how injuries occur (from running, not walking); the importance of posture, stretching, and flexibility; and what limitations you should put upon your exercise program in terms of frequency, duration, and intensity. This knowledge will be the proverbial light at the end of the tunnel for you.

If we were going to play God and build a musculoskeletal system for Adam and Eve (or Lucy), we would need some bones, ligaments, tendons, muscles, and cartilage. To put a leg together, for instance, we would take a lower-leg bone and an upper-leg bone and sandwich some cartilage between them. Cartilage is a smooth, resilient material that lets the bones slide back and forth over each other without scraping or catching. Contrary to what some people believe, the cartilage in the knee is *not* a shock absorber.

Next, we would add some ligament, which is a tough, almost nonelastic cord of muscle tissue used to lace the bones together. Once we had the bones hooked up, we would need to put the muscles on the skeleton. To attach the muscle groups to the bones, we'd need some tendons, strong, tight cords of muscle tissue.

The best-known tendon in our body is the Achilles, named after the great Greek warrior in the Trojan War. Achilles was killed when he was wounded in the heel, his one vulnerable spot, with an arrow. The Achilles tendon runs down the back of the lower-leg muscle called the calf muscle. It is the strongest in the body and connects the muscles of the calf to the bone of the heel. The rest of the limbs are assembled in approximately the same way.

Once the musculoskeletal system is all hooked up and laced together, how do we get it to move? Our big brain sends nerve impulses, much like an electrical current, down our central nervous system, called the spinal cord, and out through the nerve pathways that lead to the part or parts we want to move. These impulses cause certain muscles to contract and others to relax in a sequential order that permits us to lift a leg or scratch our nose.

As we walk, for instance, certain muscles in the leg are contracting while others are relaxing. When the contracting muscles have performed their phase of the step, they relax while the other muscles start to contract and perform *their* phase. It is easy to visualize if you think of how the strings on a marionette work. Some strings pull the leg forward while others are relaxed. Four-legged animals are put together and move in exactly the same way. There are some things evolution didn't alter. Nevertheless, millions of years before Lucy, the quadrupedal musculoskeletal system was reengineered through the long, laborious process of evolution to accommodate our unique upright bipedality. As Dr. Lovejoy explained it to me, "For bipedality to work, most of the muscle groups in the lower limbs took on new roles. These new roles in turn required changes in the muscle structure or position and, hence, in the design of the pelvis."

Dr. Lovejoy compared the human pelvis and its attached muscles with those of our closest living relative, the chimpanzee, to highlight the changes in musculoskeletal design. According to scientific analysis of deoxyribonucleic acid (DNA)—the carrier of heredity in our cells—there is a 99 percent identity between humans and chimpanzees. There is great variation in our locomotion systems, however. Chimpanzees are basically quadrupedal, whereas we are totally bipedal.

In Figure 2.2 all the corresponding muscles for the lower bodies of the chimpanzee and human are identified with their proper anatomical names. Under each name in the human illustration (Figure 2.2B) I have added its familiar name if there is one.

The need to stabilize an upright torso (as shown circled in Figure 2.1B) dictated the change of the gluteus maximus from a relatively minor muscle in the chimpanzee into the largest muscle in the human body, according to Dr. Lovejoy. The gluteus maximus is commonly referred to as the buttocks.

The gluteus maximus originates over much of the back of the pelvis and is attached to the back and side of the femur, which is the thighbone or upper-leg bone. A lot of people probably have huge rear ends because they spend too much time sitting on the biggest muscle in their body instead of using it. I can tell

FIGURE 2.2A   **FIGURE 2.2B**

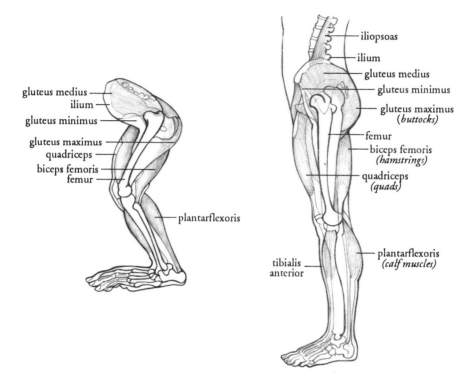

Redrawn from C. Owen Lovejoy, "Evolution of Human Walking," *Scientific American*, November 1988, pp. 118–125.

you, a good long walk every day will help remedy that problem.

Some anatomists believed the gluteus maximus served as a major propulsive muscle in upright walking, but Dr. Lovejoy disagrees: "When we walk or run, our upright trunk tends to flex forward at each foot strike, owing to momentum. The gluteus maximus has taken on the role of preventing our trunk from pitching forward. That's why it has hypertrophied [increased in size]. The gluteus maximus contribution to propulsion is limited."

There are two other gluteus muscles—medius and minimus. Unfortunately, they don't have a simple name like buttocks, and the role they play in our biped walking gait is not simple either. To explain it to me, Dr. Lovejoy deftly drew a femur, a femoral neck, and a pelvic hip socket on a pad. He was casually describing it all with terms such as "lateral flare," "fulcrum," and "gradient of stress" when my eyes crossed.

Dr. Lovejoy saw I was in trouble. So he patiently talked me through the evolutionary changes. They are remarkable; indeed, we are an unusual work of biomechanical engineering.

In the chimpanzee's leg (Figure 2.2A), you can see that the gluteus medius is just above the ilium (the top edge of the pelvis). You can reach down and feel your own ilium, which we think of as the top edge of the hipbone. The gluteus minimus and gluteus medius have two other names: anterior gluteals or abductors. Since *abductors* is one word that covers both muscles, let's stick with that. The abductors are attached near the top edge of the pelvis or hipbone and to the outside edge of the femur or upper-leg bone. Simple enough. They are two main muscles that hook the pelvis to the upper leg.

The roles these two muscles play in the locomotion system of the chimpanzee and other quadrupeds and in ours are dramatically different, however. Notice that the chimpanzee is in a crouched, contracted position. This is its normal posture. From that position the minimus and medius are powerful propulsion muscles for forward thrust and extension of the hip for speed and agility. They function the same way on a horse or a dog, which are more obvious-looking quadrupeds.

The abductors on human beings are used to keep us from tilting over when we are walking or running. This was the major evolutionary change of these muscles' function. Dr. Lovejoy explained it this way, "Imagine a head-on view of a person walking. As soon as the lead foot is placed on the ground and the trailing leg starts to swing forward, the entire body is supported on one side of the hip. Without the abductor muscles in their new role, the pelvis and trunk would tip to the unsupported side, causing rapid fatigue."

A picture is, indeed, better than a thousand words, especially when the words are engineering terms such as *fulcrum, lever arm*, and others. Figure 2.3, showing the pelvis, upper leg, and abductors, however, is something even I can understand, and it clearly shows how the abductors keep us from tilting over.

Notice how the rounded protrusion of the upper-leg bone, called the femoral head, fits into the hip socket. It functions much like a ball-and-socket trailer hitch. The abductors hook onto the top of the ilium, or hipbone, and the outside edge of the upper leg.

FIGURE 2.3

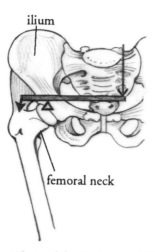

ilium

femoral neck

Redrawn from Kenneth F. Weaver, "The Search for Our Ancestors," *National Geographic*, November 1985, p. 593.

When you are standing on that leg, it is the femoral neck and head pushing into the hip socket—the fulcrum—and the pull of the powerful abductors on the thighbone that prevent your pelvis from tilting over from the weight of your torso pushing down. Whether God or evolution designed it, that is a slick piece of biomechanical engineering.

In Figure 2.3, the black triangle by the femur or femoral head is the fulcrum, the spot where the maximum compression occurs on the joint when that leg is weight-bearing. This small area is subjected to enormous amounts of pressure, causing people who have arthritis in this joint to suffer greatly. Lucy did not have to worry about arthritis, however; she didn't live long enough. Most australopithecines didn't live longer than 20 to 30 years.

Although chimpanzees are quadrupeds, they can walk upright for short distances, but they tire quickly because of their pelvic structure and gluteal muscle positioning. The November 1985 issue of *National Geographic* had a cover story called "The Search for Early Man." It traced our development from Lucy to *Homo sapiens* and showed little Lucy and a chimpanzee in an upright walking mode (see Figure 2.4).

The chimpanzee (Figure 2.4B) tilts with each step to position its body over its foot for support, whereas Lucy (Figure 2.4A) is upright. Her foot passes under her body as she walks in a less

FIGURE 2.4A   FIGURE 2.4B

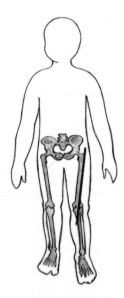
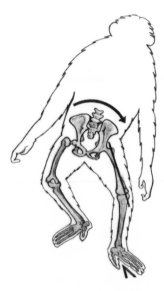

fatiguing manner. Her different pelvic structure and thighbone attachment at the hip by the gluteal muscles conclusively prove that Lucy was the start of something special—the human species.

Another major muscle that took on a new role in the evolution of our walking gait is the biceps femoris, one of the group of three known to all of us as the hamstrings. These are the big muscles that run up the back of our upper leg and attach to the pelvis. In the chimpanzee, they serve as powerful hip extensors for forward thrust and contribute more to propulsion than the gluteal muscles do.

In bipedal walking, the hamstrings don't extend the limb to propel the body forward; instead, they act as a brake, to stop the leg at the end of its forward swing. The human leg is a long, heavy pendulum, and when it swings forward it takes powerful muscles to bring it to a halt. That is the hamstrings' job.

The logical question, then, is, If the hamstrings stop the leg swing, what gets the leg swing started? It seems that the laws of physics and gravity are aided by a muscle called the iliopsoas (pronounced ill-e-ó-so-as; the *p* is silent). It doesn't have a user-friendly synonym, so that's it. (*Iliopsoas* is not in my dictionaries or my medical encyclopedia.)

Perhaps the reason the iliopsoas is so unpublicized is that it is positioned to do its job with very little risk of injury. Have you ever heard of anybody who had a pain in the iliopsoas? Me neither. You can see in Figure 2.3 that the iliopsoas lies along the bottom of the spinal column. It originates deep in the pelvis and extends forward to an attachment point on the upper leg.

Dr. Lovejoy explained its function this way: "The leg swing starts when the toe of the trailing limb leaves the ground. Like a pendulum at one end of its arc, gravity pulls it toward the other direction, and the iliopsoas gives the limb a tug forward to speed up the swing to the other end of its arc, where the hamstrings contract to decelerate and stop the swing. When the leg swing stops, you plant your heel, and the process reverses itself with the other leg." It worked the same way for Lucy 3 million years ago.

Generally we don't think of the leg as a pendulum, but in fact legs and arms are both pendulums. According to Dr. Lovejoy, they are *compound pendulums*, which calls for a bit of explanation. Compound pendulums are like two pendulums in one. For instance, if you stand on one leg with your other leg stiff and straight at the knee and your foot off the floor, that leg will swing from the hip socket, just like a pendulum. Now sit in a chair, with your upper leg resting on the chair bottom and the foot of that leg slightly off the floor. Your lower leg, which is hinged at the knee, will now swing back and forth like a pendulum. That is a compound pendulum.

The arms are also hinged to be compound pendulums. With your arm hanging straight down at your side and rigid at the elbow, you can swing it back and forth from the shoulder like a long pendulum. Now hold your upper arm out so that your elbow is shoulder high. The lower arm, hinged at the elbow, freely swings back and forth—two pendulums in one.

In Chapters 5 and 6, when you learn the biomechanics of the various walking intensities, you will see how the arm pendulums and leg pendulums interrelate. Not only do they counterbalance the normal walking gait, but, because they have the compound feature, they can be manipulated to help you walk at the speed of a jogger, to burn more calories, and develop a higher fitness level—maybe to even become a race walker if you have a competitive urge.

The waitress at the Pufferbelly was clearing away the dinner dishes when I glanced at my watch; an enjoyable and very edu-

FIGURE 2.5A   2.5B   2.5C   2.5D

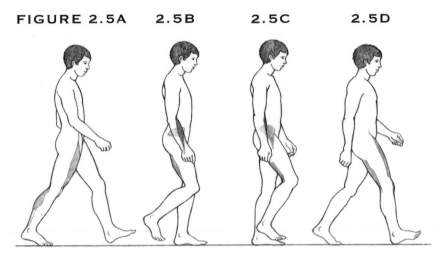

Redrawn from C. Owen Lovejoy, "Evolution of Human Walking," *Scientific American*, November 1988, pp. 118–125.

cational two hours had just whistled by in what seemed like five minutes. I ordered tea, Dr. Lovejoy ordered coffee, and his class of one resumed. "In human beings the demands of stabilizing the upright pelvis and controlling the leg swing occupy several muscle groups that serve for propulsion in the chimpanzee and other quadrupeds. Only two muscle groups, the quadriceps and the plantarflexors, are left in positions that enable them to produce a ground reaction or propulsion effect."

This last sentence sounds more complicated than it is. As Figure 2.2B shows, the quadriceps are the big muscles—a group of four—on the front of the upper leg. Many exercisers refer to them as *quads*. They end in the stout patellar tendon, which crosses the kneecap and is anchored to the tibia, the large main bone of the lower leg. If your knee is bent, this muscle group contracts to straighten it.

The plantarflexors are known to everyone as the calf muscles. They originate at the back of the lower leg and are attached to the heel by the Achilles tendon. Remember when you rotated your ankle with both feet under you and you went straight up, ending up on your toes like a ballet dancer? Your calf muscles were the power behind this move.

Figure 2.5 puts all the bones, tendons, and major muscles of the walking gait to work. If you take a full step, you can see the sequence of muscle activity required to propel you forward.

Figure 2.5A has the weight-bearing right leg angled behind the body, ready to push off with the toes as the calf muscle contracts and causes the ankle to rotate. At the same time, the quads on the front of the thigh contract to straighten the knee. The foot pushing against the ground propels the body forward. The right foot leaves the ground when the heel of the left foot is planted to stop the falling torso. Most people don't normally think of walking as a lifting and falling action. You can clearly see, however, that, as one leg is pushing from behind, you would fall forward on your face without the benefit of another leg swinging forward to stop your falling body.

Figure 2.5B has the left leg weight-bearing. Gravity has caused the right leg to start to swing forward, and the iliopsoas muscle gives it a tug to speed its swing. In Figures 2.5B and 2.5C, the hamstrings contract to flex the leg slightly at the knee so that the foot will clear the ground as it swings under the body. This demonstrates the use of our leg's compound pendulum feature.

Figure 2.5D shows that near the end of the forward leg swing the quadricep muscles contract again to straighten the knee before the heel is planted. The hamstrings contract to decelerate and ultimately stop the leg swing. The left leg is now angled behind the body and pushes off as the calf muscles contract. A complete step has been taken, and it has used *all* the major muscle groups in the lower body—just what you want for an effective exercise.

In comparing our bipedality with Lucy's, Dr. Lovejoy said: "In one respect Lucy seems to have been even better designed for bipedality than we are. The reason lies in the accelerated growth of the human brain during the past 3 million years and the change in the modern human pelvis." Flipping over a fresh page on the pad, he sketched an approximate version of Lucy's pelvis, abductors, and hip socket. Unfortunately, we were back to some heavy engineering terms—*lever arms, cantilevered beams,* and so on. I found it fascinating, but I am sure you would nod off on me if I tried to give it all to you verbatim.

Briefly, it goes like this: the ilium, or top hip edge, on the modern female (Figure 2.6A) is more contracted than on Lucy (Figure 2.6B). It is less elliptical and more rounded. It was this feature, combined with the hip socket, femoral neck, and abductor muscle attachments that gave Lucy a biomechanical walking advantage over us, according to Dr. Lovejoy. She was simply better engineered at this critical joint.

FIGURE 2.6A

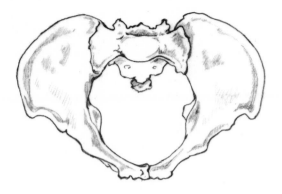

FIGURE 2.6B

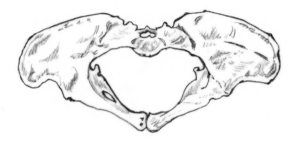

Redrawn from C. Owen Lovejoy, "Evolution of Human Walking," *Scientific American*, November 1988, pp. 118–125.

Figure 2.6 is drawings from photographs of top views of the pelvises. You can readily see the expansion of the birth canal that also occurred because of the increase in brain size in the 3 million years since Lucy.

Lucy's birth canal was wide but short from front to back. "This constriction was tolerable because her infant's cranium would have been no larger than a baby chimpanzee's," Dr. Lovejoy explained. He explained the change this way: "As human ancestors evolved a larger brain, the pelvic opening had to become rounder. The pelvis had to expand from front to back, but, at the same time, it contracted slightly from side to side." As a result, two important changes occurred: "The flare of the ilia was reduced, leaving us with a somewhat shorter abductor lever arm. Meanwhile, the head of the femur became enlarged to withstand increased pressure from the harder-working abductors."

Let's see if I can translate that into everyday language. *Ilia* is plural for the ilium, or hip edges, on each side of the pelvis. The "head of the femur" is shown in Figure 2.3. This resembles the ball on a trailer hitch, and it fits into the hip socket. The "harder-working abductors" are the hip muscles in Figures 2.2B and 2.3 (our old friends gluteus minimus and gluteus medius). In simple terms, then, Lucy had a biomechanical advantage over us because her pelvis was shaped so that the hip socket, femoral neck, and abductor muscle attachments were stronger and more efficient. "These changes are less pronounced in the modern male pelvis, where the abductors retain some of their former mechanical advantage," Dr. Lovejoy pointed out. Maybe this is because we lucky males don't need a birth canal and are spared the pain of childbirth.

That pain is partly the result of humans' unique ability to walk upright. "The difficulty of accommodating an effective bipedal hip joint for walking and running and an adequate passage for a large infant brain remains acute, and the human birth process is one of the most difficult in the animal kingdom," Dr. Lovejoy explained. "The process of birth in Lucy and her contemporaries would have been more complex than in a chimpanzee but much easier than the modern human birth process."

Figure 2.7 compares the pelvic structure and birth canal (shown from the back) of a chimpanzee (A), Lucy (B), and modern woman (C). In explaining these illustrations to me, Dr. Lovejoy pointed out, "The birth process has *competed* with bipedality in shaping the modern human pelvis." In the chimpanzee pelvis, which is noticeably different from both Lucy's and modern woman's, the head of the fetus descends without difficulty through the inlet (top), midplane (middle), and outlet (bottom) of the large birth canal.

"In Lucy," Dr. Lovejoy said, "notice that the birth process was somewhat more difficult. Her birth canal was broad but constricted from front to back. Her infant's cranium could pass through only if it was first turned sideways and then tilted."

Human birth is even more complex, according to Dr. Lovejoy.

FIGURE 2.7A   FIGURE 2.7B   FIGURE 2.7C

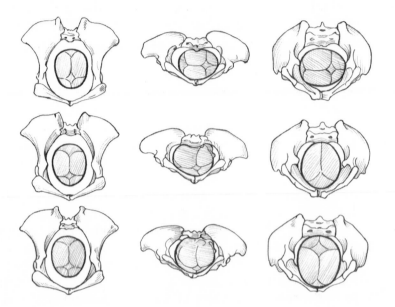

Redrawn from C. Owen Lovejoy, "Evolution of Human Walking," *Scientific American*, November 1988, pp. 118–125.

"The much larger brain in the human infant demands a rounder birth canal. Even with the rounder birth canal, the human birth process is complex and traumatic, requiring a second rotation of the fetal cranium within the birth canal."

By now, it is obvious why Dr. Lovejoy said he would like to get his hands on a 6-million-year-old pelvis. The pelvis is the pivotal part of the human anatomy that makes our upright walking gait possible.

Unfortunately Dr. Lovejoy may have a long wait. According to *National Geographic*'s 1985 "Early Man" story, none of the primate fossils before *Australopithecus afarensis* (Lucy) has been complete enough to be accepted by the scientific community as a human ancestor. The article stated, "Until more fossils—and more complete specimens—are found, the long geologic epoch known as the Miocene [25 million to 10 million years ago] will remain a largely veiled chapter in hominid evolution." For now, little Lucy is our first known bipedal walker.

It seems entirely appropriate that our oldest example of the walking gait is a female. Women make up almost two thirds of the exercise walkers in the United States, and, in the hundreds of clinics I have conducted over the past five years, they tell me in a resounding chorus that walking is their favorite exercise. Rightly so. Women are natural walkers; their walking gait is definitely more fluid and rhythmic than men's. I know of numerous husbands who can't keep up with their wives. My gender may resent that, but it is indisputably true.

Lucy's pelvis clearly differentiates her from apes and chimpanzees. Dr. Lovejoy said, "The rest of her skeleton reveals equally dramatic modifications that favor bipedality and rule out other modes of locomotion." For example, "The knee is adapted for withstanding greater stress during complete extension [fully straightened] than the knee of other primates." According to Dr. Lovejoy, the knee design brings the femur (upper leg) and tibia (big bone of the lower leg) together at a slight angle, so the foot can easily be planted directly under the body's center of mass when the body weight is supported on one leg. The ankle is also modified for supporting the entire body weight. In addition, he said, "A shock-absorbing arch helps the foot to cope with the added load."

To remove any doubt about whether Lucy was part ape, Dr. Lovejoy pointed out, "The great toe is no longer opposable as it is in quadrupedal apes, but runs parallel to the other toes [see Figure 2.4]. The foot is now a propulsive lever for upright walking, rather than a grasping device for arboreal travel." He added, "The arms have also become less suited to climbing: both the limb as a whole and the fingers have grown shorter than they are in the apes." End of class.

The warm late afternoon had given way to night, and a cool rain was falling as we stood in the entryway at the Pufferbelly. My class on anthropology, human anatomy, locomotion, and biomechanics had lasted almost four hours. I regretted that I couldn't sign up for a whole semester. As we shook hands in farewell, Dr. Lovejoy said reassuringly, "Casey, you can state in your book without any reservations that the bipedal human walking gait is at least 3 million years old. Not only was Lucy capable of walking upright; it had become her only choice."

When I got to my car, I sat there for a few minutes to let these words sink in. What a frightful predicament for Lucy! When she emerged from the primeval mists that shroud the beginning of life on earth, she was small, frail, and vulnerable. She had given up the ability to find food and safety in the arboreal world of her distant cousins. She was born a million years before even the most primitive stone tools. To move about for food, safety, and survival, Lucy relied mainly on her ability to walk and run. She could not run very fast, however, compared with the quadrupedal carnivorous predators with whom she shared her world.

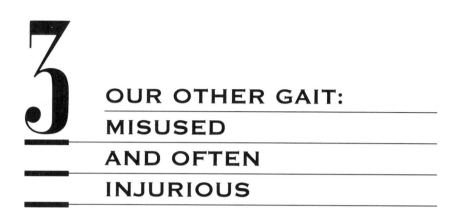

3

OUR OTHER GAIT: MISUSED AND OFTEN INJURIOUS

Most people who have a fear of flying generally defend their fear with the line "If God had meant humans to fly, He would have given us wings." To paraphrase this maxim as it applies to running, I believe that if God had meant humans to run, He would have given us the locomotion system of a horse. He surely would not have made us upright and two-legged.

As an injured exercise runner, I will tell you that I would never have run that first step if I had known as much about walking then as I do now. This chapter will be informative for you because it will help you to learn how your running gait functions in relation to your walking gait. You will also become aware of how vastly overpublicized, overrated, and overprescribed exercise running has been, and to some extent still is. I guarantee that you will take up walking with more confidence, pride, and determination when you find out that the *only* thing running can give you that walking doesn't is injury! You will become a believer and will spread the word.

Walking has always been the entry-level, wimp exercise for the obese and unfit, or for older people, like me. That's where everybody is supposed to start and then graduate to the macho, intense exercise called jogging, running, or whatever. Having been an exercise runner for three years before my right knee gave out, I can tell you that there was not one time that I truly enjoyed running as much as I do my daily walks. To me exercise running was always a jarring, boring, no-brainer exercise.

WHY RUNNING CAUSES INJURIES

Having said that, however, I have to admit that running helped me lose 25 pounds and develop an excellent fitness level. So what's the beef? Injury! But don't take my word for it. The cover of the February 1991 issue of *Runner's World* reads "Complete Injury Prevention Program at Last!" The opening paragraph of the story stated: "During the course of any year, you have a fifty-fifty chance of developing a running injury that will alter or stop your training. In other words, each year 50 percent of all runners, from recreational athletes to elite, sustain an injury that affects their running."

The article was written by a doctor, who said: "One of the best things any runner can do to prevent injury is to follow a regular stretching and strengthening program." This may help some, but probably not much. As you learned in the last chapter, becoming upright placed our center of mass on *top* of our propulsion system. Unlike that of a quadruped, our musculoskeletal system takes a pounding from running, which predictably leads to injury—even in people who don't run very much.

For instance, in the November 1990 issue of *Fit News*, published by the American Running and Fitness Association, a study of 300 male infantry trainees at Ft. Benning in Georgia was cited. The men were divided into two companies. One company ran 60 miles during 12 weeks of training, while the other ran 130 miles. The injury rate was 33 percent in the low-mileage company and 42 percent in the 130-mile group. Ages were not given, but we can assume that a peacetime volunteer infantry trainee is in his teens or twenties.

A 33 percent injury rate for young men who only ran 60 miles in 12 weeks (5.0 miles per week) indicates that running as an exercise is seriously flawed. A 42 percent injury rate for the other group, who only averaged 10.8 miles per week, is a pitiful statistic for a physical activity that is supposed to contribute to fitness, health, and well-being. Injury is the most frequent reason people give for dropping out of an exercise program. Once you understand how running works biomechanically as your secondary gait of locomotion, you will never use it as your primary exercise.

The evolutionary process that gave little Lucy her unique walking gait also altered her running gait. Dr. Lovejoy's observation "When we became upright we lost speed and agility" was not just a random remark. When we evolved from quadruped to biped, we lost the powerful forward thrust of hind legs. The body's center of mass is out in front of the propulsion muscles of a quadruped. The center of mass on a human is on top of the propulsion muscles, as shown in Figure 2.1B. This means that, with every running step we take, our entire body weight lands on a single foot that stops our falling body and then propels us upward and forward for the next step.

Exercise physiologists calculate that we land with the force of 3 to 4 times our body weight. The figure 3.5 is generally accepted. Therefore a 200-pound man lands with the force of 700 pounds on each foot with each running step. This force is transmitted up the leg to the pelvis and lower back. Our musculoskeletal system does not have shock absorbers to handle such an impact. Something has to give—and over time it usually does. The history of runners with stress fractures, shinsplints, knee, hip, and lower-back injuries is well documented. You only have to look at how we are constructed compared with a quadruped to realize that we are not built for prolonged running.

The evolutionary role of running in all animals has been as a fight-or-flight survival gait to be used in short spurts. In today's wild animal kingdom, running is used only as a survival gait. Dr. Lovejoy said he doesn't know of any animal that runs more than 3 minutes at a time in its natural environment. If you have watched any of the fine shows about African wildlife on public television, at some time you have probably seen a lioness chasing a zebra. She is running for her lunch, and the zebra is running for its life. The chase is brief. If the lioness doesn't bring down the zebra in a short run, she pulls up and looks for a slower one. The chase does not go on mile after mile, day after day; consequently, neither animal suffers injury from running.

Humans injure not only themselves from prolonged running but also, sometimes, other animals. Of all the thoroughbred foals born each year, only about 50 percent survive training. Those that make it to the races often have brief careers. In a horse race, at the point of fatigue, generally in the stretch, when the horse naturally wants to slow down, the 110-pound jockey on its back starts whipping it. Many horses suffer injury when forced to run in a state of fatigue, just as human athletes lose coordination and tend to suffer injuries when tired.

Stress fractures are a rarity among dogs except in racing greyhounds. They are raced frequently for pari-mutuel wagering. Consequently, they suffer stress fractures that they would not experience in a natural setting. Stress fractures are common in human runners. In the "Questions from Readers, Answers from Experts" section of the November 1986 issue of *Runner's World*, a reader with a stress fracture asked for advice.

The magazine's expert, a doctor, answered: "A runner gets a stress fracture when repetitive pounding and muscular action on the leg exceed the strength and reparative capacity of the bone. While an acute fracture is the result of a single traumatic event, a stress fracture happens because of repeated, less severe stresses over a period of time. . . . Stress fractures are found in only two other species—the racehorse and the racing greyhound—and then only when the animals have been forced to run under human supervision." He added, "It looks like we are the only ones too stubborn to heed pain's clear warnings."

Why don't horses suffer stress fractures when in a natural setting? The March 1988 issue of *Equine Sportsmedicine News* explained how early horses moved about without human intervention: "The ancestor of today's highly regimented equine roamed the plains and forests freely, rarely staying in one spot long enough for the muscles to get stiff. He kept one ear to the wind so as to stay ahead of his predators, through continuous movement or short bursts of trotting. Running at top speed from a standstill was not part of his usual activity." And we call them *dumb* animals?

If running carries the excess baggage of injury, how did it achieve such wide acceptance as an exercise for humans? Running for exercise was launched fifteen years ago, when Jim Fixx's *The Complete Book of Running* was published. Fixx's book was extremely well-written and inspirational to the point that if you didn't like running you tended to question your normality. Luckily, the adversity of my knee injury forced me to adopt walking as an exercise, or I might still be slogging up and down the road wondering why I was feeling miserable instead of elated.

Jim Fixx took a sport and made it appealing as a mass exercise. Until his book, most people viewed running as a spectator sport at high school, college, and Olympic track and field events. Yes, there were some exercise runners before Fixx, but as a percentage of the population they were few. Athletes who run in track events frequently suffer injuries, but it is considered part of the sport. Mary Decker Slaney, perhaps the best woman runner of the past decade, spent about half of her career healing from injuries. The running career of Alberto Salazar, the great American marathoner, was over before he was 30 because of injuries.

Injury is accepted, of course, in every sport as part of the risk of the participant. If Mike Ditka, the popular coach of the Chicago Bears, wrote an inspirational book about football as a way for the general public to lose weight and get fit, would anyone be surprised when a rash of knee injuries, concussions, and broken limbs occurred? Running at track and field events is a great spectator sport. As a mass exercise, however, running's role must be redefined.

It is apparent that we are misusing the running gait when we employ it for prolonged periods for exercise. *Misuse* is a different word from the one exercise physiologists and proponents of running use. They say most running injuries result from *overuse*. It will be easy, however, for you to understand why *misuse* is more appropriate than *overuse* for running injuries by comparing our biomechanical locomotion system with a mechanical locomotion system, such as that of a pickup truck. If a businessman or farmer bought a half-ton pickup truck and continually overloaded it with three to five tons, he would experience broken springs, bent axles, and a variety of other mechanical failures. The truck has certain performance limitations engineered into it. Similarly, our locomotion system is biomechanically engineered for the performance of unlimited walking but limited running. The breakdown of the truck is predictable; so is injury to an exercise runner. The problem of injuries from prolonged running is clearly *misuse*, not overuse.

Putting injury aside for the moment, exercise running is less desirable than walking because it is not as effective for caloric expenditure and aerobic fitness as we have been taught. The research that sheds new light on this point comes from zoologists, not exercise physiologists. Zoologists have found that when any animal—including the human animal—runs, it conserves energy for the speed it is traveling.

I know that probably doesn't sound right, but stay with me. Only the human animal runs deliberately merely to burn energy, and that is a fairly recent phenomenon.

Up until now, most of the information about exercise running has trickled down from its sports application, as a track and field event. Anyone who ran a 10K race (6.2 miles) or a marathon (26 miles, 385 yards) had to be aerobically fit and obviously used a lot of energy. Thus it followed that if all of us ran up and down the road for exercise, we would get fit and use a lot of energy. This is undeniably true, but zoological research on animals' gaits of locomotion—including ours—conclusively proves that running doesn't use as much energy as we once thought. If this is the case, then the primary reason that people jog and run is, if not totally eliminated, drastically reduced. It was the research and considerate help of a zoologist in England and a zoologist at Harvard that helped me sort this out.

GAIT EFFICIENCY

The voice was crisp, businesslike, and British, but with a very accommodating tone: "Yes, I'll be glad to gather up copies of my research that I have here in my office and send them off to you right away." I offered to send a check to cover copying costs and postage but was firmly turned down. "That won't be necessary; those of us working in research rely on the cooperation of others all the time. I have often made similar requests. Let me know if I can be of further help, and good luck with your book."

I had called R. McNeill Alexander, a professor of zoology at the University of Leeds in England, and, through the miracle of the transatlantic direct-dial system, he sounded as close as my grocer. Four days later a large manila envelope arrived with eight research papers on walking and running as gaits of locomotion in bipeds and quadrupeds. It also contained this note: "I am sorry that this is a very incomplete selection: I am out of copies of other papers that you might like to have." It was everything I needed, however, and someday I am going to England to thank Professor Alexander in person.

Before walking and running became exercises or sports, they were—and still are—simply the two gaits of locomotion of the human biped and of all our ancestors back to and before Lucy. However, in the past few decades in Western industrialized countries, walking and running have been utilized for premeditated exercise to make up for the loss of regular physical activity caused by our sedentary life-styles.

Running has been most widely recommended to produce the highest level of aerobic and cardiovascular fitness. It is also considered to burn the most calories in the least time. For example, in the February 1987 issue of *The Runner* magazine, a medical expert wrote, "Running, of course, is more strenuous than walking and provides greater cardiovascular benefits." He also stated: "Most fitness buffs would agree in terms of exercise satisfaction, walking can't keep up with running." Wrong on both counts.

To get another perspective on running versus walking as an exercise, I checked the library at the Institute for Aerobics Research and found a book entitled *Jog, Run, Race*. Flipping through the pages to "Lesson 5," entitled "Introducing Walking" (which was all of one and a half pages), I read the author's attitude of disdain: "It isn't an admission of defeat to start with walking." How could walking ever be considered an "admission of defeat"? Unfortunately, that's how most runners view it.

The total extent of the author's walking instruction is "This is the type of walking I propose for the first month: make no big deal of it. Follow no formal plan, do no special preparations for it, and buy no special equipment. Just start walking." This author is only repeating the same old condescending line that all running proponents have been putting out ad nauseam. Lesson 7, entitled "Speed Up," says: "Your persistence and patience are about to be rewarded. This month you *step up* to running" (my emphasis). Before this chapter is over, and most assuredly by the end of this book, you will find that running is no "step up." For most exercisers, running is the wrong step.

The most common misinformation about walking is delivered in Lesson 9, entitled "Introducing Jogging." The author writes: "Jogging and running never need to take much time because they are fast acting exercises. To draw the same physical benefits from a jog or run as you get from a walk, you need only about a fourth as much time. In other words, the effects of an hour's walk can be had in a 15 minute jog-run." This is the gospel that has been preached by most runners and exercise experts over the years. Unfortunately, many still do preach it, and they are wrong.

The reason for this common error is that walking is viewed as an exercise instead of in its role as our primary gait of locomotion. It was during the research for my first book, *Aerobic Walking*, that I stumbled onto some zoological research by Professor C. Richard Taylor of the Museum of Comparative Zoology at Har-

FIGURE 3.1A   **FIGURE 3.1B**

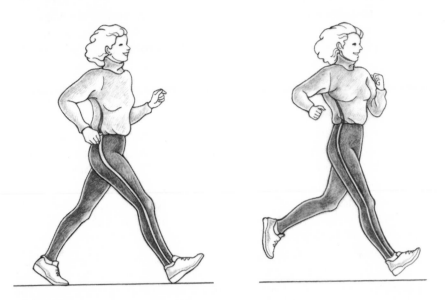

vard University on animals' gaits of locomotion and why animals change gaits. This research convinced me that exercise physiologists were ignoring the most important variable between walking and running—*gait efficiency*.

Back in July 1985, I traveled to Harvard and talked to Professor Taylor about his research. He and others have proven that human running uses much less energy than might be expected. Once this point is scientifically established, running for exercise becomes less desirable and certainly not a "step up."

As explained in the last chapter, walking is the lifting and falling of our body as the trailing foot pushes off against the ground and the lead leg swings forward and becomes the support and weight-bearing limb. As compound pendulums, the legs have a natural arc-and-swing frequency; hence, walking is mechanical. When you break into a run, however, you shift (literally) from mechanical pendulum action to the elastic action of muscles and tendons.

The two critical phases that distinguish walking from running are shown in Figure 3.1. The walker (A) is in the *double-stance phase*, the brief moment when the front heel is planted and before the back foot leaves the ground. The *flight phase* of a runner (B)

is just the opposite. Instead of both feet being on the ground before
the trailing limb starts forward, both feet are off the ground.

Simply stated, a walker has at least one foot on the ground at
all times, and there is a brief period when both feet are in contact
with the ground. Conversely, a runner has a phase in which both
feet are off the ground simultaneously and never has more than
one foot in contact with the ground at any time. Whether you are
going slow or fast, or whether it is called a jog or a run, once both
feet leave the ground, you have shifted to your running gait and
are using elastic energy in much the way that a bouncing ball does.

You have shifted gaits many times, but you probably didn't
realize exactly why. I am sure there have been occasions when you
were late for an appointment and were walking at a pretty fast
pace, then you reached a point at which it was much easier to run
slowly than to walk faster. That's when you shifted from the mechanical walk to the elastic run.

Once you shift to a run, you are *using less energy (burning fewer
calories) and less oxygen than if you had increased your speed by
walking*. Please read this again and again and again! Most people
don't believe it. Nevertheless, zoological locomotion research dis-
proves the old wives' tale that running is superior to walking for
weight loss and aerobic fitness—or for any reason involving exercise.

For more than a decade Professor Alexander has been concerned
with applying the principles of engineering mechanics to the study
of animal and human locomotion systems. He is the author of a
number of books, including *Animal Mechanics*. The material Professor Alexander sent me explains how our two gaits function
biomechanically. When we went from quadruped to biped, we not
only lost speed and agility, but also lost a gait. We can walk and
run, but a quadruped can walk, *trot*, and run. I know baseball
announcers frequently say that a player "trots down to first base"
after being walked. He may run slowly, but he doesn't trot; only
quadrupeds can do that.

In a research paper published in *American Scientist* in 1984,
Professor Alexander stated: "Most mammals the size of cats and
larger walk and run using the same mechanical principles as in the
corresponding human gaits. A cat or horse walking is essentially
similar to two people walking, one behind the other." In explaining
the trot Alexander said: "A quadrupedal mammal trotting is like

two people running, one behind the other." The running quadruped has a tremendous advantage over the running human biped. Not only does the quadruped have its center of mass in front of the propulsion muscles for greater forward thrust, but its large back muscles also contribute to the power of its run.

To explain the elastic properties of muscles and tendons, Professor Alexander used the example of a rubber ball and a pogo stick in a paper entitled "Human Walking and Running," published in the *Journal of Biological Education*. When a ball is bounced on the ground, it compresses and flattens on the bottom. "When a ball is squashed, elastic strain energy is stored in the deformed rubber. This energy can be recovered in an elastic recoil. The same effect is achieved with steel springs instead of rubber in the toy called a pogo stick."

A person running, then, is much like a bouncing ball or a child on a pogo stick. According to Professor Alexander, "Muscles and tendons in the leg store the elastic strain energy at each footfall and it is released as the foot leaves the ground." The elastic strain energy of running significantly reduces our energy requirements. Professor Alexander explained: "This is how metabolic energy requirements are reduced to less than half of what would otherwise be needed." Running is nature's most efficient gait.

All the solid materials in the leg have some elastic properties and must to some extent act as energy stores. However, Professor Alexander pointed out: "The skeleton is too stiff to be deformed much by the forces that act in running, so it cannot store much elastic strain energy. . . . The muscles and their tendons seem likely to be much more important. . . . It is probable that in running most of the elastic strain energy is stored in the tendons."

The suggestion that tendons serve as springs may seem surprising, but Professor Alexander explained it this way: "[The] tendon can do so because, although it cannot be stretched much, it is very strong and can store a great deal of elastic-strain energy." As an example, "Experiments in which sheep tendons were stretched in imitation of running . . . showed that 93 percent of the work done stretching them could be recovered in an elastic recoil." As a comparison, "This is about as good as the best rubbers." Thus, exercise runners bounce along in nature's most efficient gait using elastic strain energy.

Here is an excellent description of how elastic energy is used in running: "During the early part of the stance phase, the muscles,

FIGURE 3.2

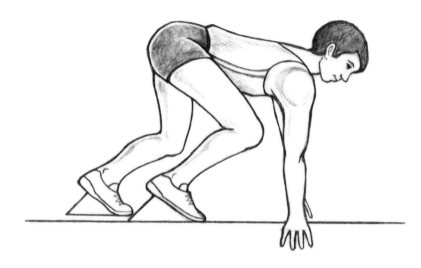

ligaments, and tendons absorb concussion by stretching. As they stretch, they store energy which is released at a later stage in the stance phase to aid in propulsion. Recovery of this 'rebound' energy from the tendon and ligament springs is an energy-saving mechanism." It is interesting that this is quoted not from *Runner's World* but from the April 1987 issue of *Equine Sportsmedicine News*. The muscles and tendons in a running horse function exactly like those in a human. Evolution didn't change this part of our locomotion system.

But even though our running gait is energy-efficient, like that of other animals, we are slowpokes as runners. Commenting on our physical makeup, Professor Alexander stated: "Our legs and feet are rather like those of our tree climbing ancestors, much less specialized for running than in many other mammals. Consequently, we are rather slow." For comparative running times, he said, "A good human sprinter will race 100 meters in about 10 seconds at a speed of 22 MPH. . . . Most horse and greyhound races, however, are won at speeds between 34 to 38 MPH." We think the human world record of 3 minutes, 46.3 seconds for the mile is fast, but the world record for a thoroughbred horse over the same distance is 1 minute, 32⅕ seconds.

An interesting example of a human trying to capture the horizontal thrust of a quadruped is shown in Figure 3.2. The sprinter gets a strong horizontal push against the ground and the starting

FIGURE 3.3

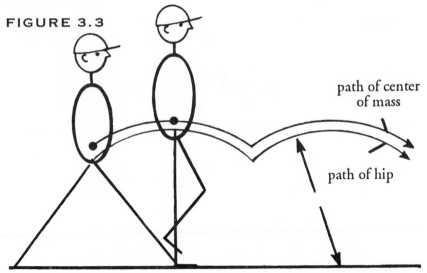

path of center
of mass

path of hip

blocks, but in a couple of strides the body is upright again and the running disadvantages of human biped locomotion return.

The biomechanics of the walking gait can best be seen in animated Figure 3.3, which shows that the center of mass (the black dot) is at its lowest point when both feet are on the ground. As the trunk of the body passes over the weight-bearing leg, the center of mass is at its highest point. It then begins to fall as the weight-bearing leg becomes the trailing leg.

You can see that walking involves an alternate rising and falling of the body. It also involves alternate braking and accelerating; as the front foot stops the body from falling, the back foot pushes the body forward. This all works smoothly, and you are probably not conscious of the rising, falling, decelerating, accelerating activity that is involved with each step cycle.

It works very smoothly, that is, until you start to walk very fast. As you accelerate, however, you reach a point at which it is simply more convenient to switch from your mechanical gait—walking—to your elastic gait—running. Other animals do so for the same reason you do: it is easier and *more energy efficient* for faster speed.

A horse in a field may be walking along and then start to trot. After it trots a way, it may break into a full run. It went through all three of its gaits, but how did it know exactly when to move from one gait to the next? That question was answered in a study by Professors Taylor of Harvard and Donald F. Hoyt of California State Polytechnic University. Their study has a direct bearing on whether it makes more sense to walk or to run for exercise.

Interestingly, the results of the study showed that the horse shifts to a faster gait for the same reason that we humans shift to a faster gait: to conserve energy as speed increases. Taylor and Hoyt trained three small horses to walk, trot, and run on a motorized treadmill. They reported: "Using measurements of rates of oxygen consumption as an indicator of rates of energy consumption, we have confirmed that the natural gait at any speed, indeed, entails the smallest possible energy expenditure." This is true for humans as well.

Here is the part of the study that I believe is most important to an exerciser. Professors Taylor and Hoyt taught their horses to extend their gaits. By this I mean that when the horses would normally go from a walk to a trot, they taught them to walk faster. Further, when the horses would normally go from a trot to a run, they taught them to trot faster. Professor Taylor called this the "extended gait." Taylor and Hoyt wrote: "When the gaits were extended beyond their normal range of speeds, oxygen consumption was *higher* in the extended gait than in that which the animal would normally be using." Very important! If as an exerciser you want to use more oxygen to burn more calories, which calls for a higher heart rate to pump the oxygenated blood to the muscles, don't go from a walk to a run; instead, simply extend your walking gait and walk faster.

Gaits of locomotion have striking functional similarities to mechanical gears. One way to understand the biomechanics of gait efficiency is to compare it to gear efficiency in an automobile. Anyone who can drive a manual-transmission car will understand immediately. For instance, if two cars are traveling side by side at 60 miles per hour and one is in third gear and the other in fifth gear, the one in third gear will burn more fuel and have a faster engine speed (more revolutions per minute) than the one in fifth. Thus, at 60 miles per hour, fifth gear is more efficient. Higher gears are used for higher speeds.

Gait efficiency in humans and other animals works the same way. If a walker and a jogger exercise side by side at an 11-minute-mile pace, for instance, the walker will burn more calories, use more oxygen, and have a higher heart rate than the jogger because the walking gait at that speed is very *inefficient*; it requires more energy. The purpose of exercise is to use energy. Thus, the walker gets better exercise results (cardiovascular fitness and weight control) than does the jogger, without any of the jarring impact or high rate of injury that joggers and runners suffer.

The application of the information developed in this study helps to establish walking as the most injury-free, sustainable, effective, and complete exercise. We all walk every day, but over the past two decades of the fitness boom we have been led to believe that walking is of limited value, especially for those who want an intensive aerobic exercise or who want to burn the most calories in the least time.

Most exercise experts view a brisk 15-minute mile as the maximum pace for exercise walkers. It is at about this pace or a little faster, however, that people shift their gait into a run. That is the opposite of what you should do, and in Chapter 6 you will learn how to extend your walking gait to get the fitness of a runner without the injury that goes with running.

According to conventional wisdom, the primary reason to run for exercise is that walking lacks the intensity to elevate the heart rate to the aerobic training range, which in turn increases aerobic capacity, which in turn increases cardiovascular fitness and caloric expenditure. But conventional wisdom is sometimes wrong.

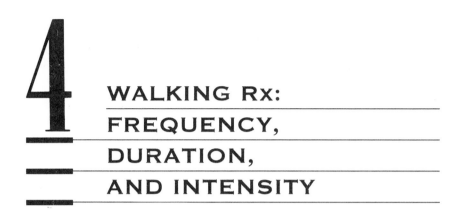

4
WALKING Rx: FREQUENCY, DURATION, AND INTENSITY

God, fate, and luck seem to influence the events in most of our lives, and there are rare occasions when you are certain that all three are working for you. Such was a day for me in early August 1988. I was on the morning trail ride at the beautiful C-Lazy-U Ranch in the mountains outside Granby, Colorado, with a friend of twenty years, Dolph Bridgewater. As we were winding our way through an aspen grove, Bridgewater asked if I had brought a copy of my book, *Aerobic Walking*, to the ranch. He said he wanted to read it. I laughed and said I had a case of them in the trunk of my car; would one be enough? I am always prepared to sell the benefits of walking, particularly to guys like Bridgewater, who is a runner.

Bridgewater is chairman of the Brown Group, Inc., in St. Louis, Missouri, which owns the Brown Shoe Company—best known for Buster Brown shoes for kids and Naturalizer shoes for women. His company was just starting to make a woman's exercise-walking shoe, and he wanted my views on the future of exercise walking. As a result of that conversation on the riding trail, I became the walking consultant for Naturalizer's NaturalSport Shoe Division. I was comfortably retired and frankly didn't want a job. I was convinced, however, that there was a glaring need for two walking studies: one that would prove aerobic walking is as effective for aerobic exercise and weight loss as running, and another that would prove aerobic walking can be used as a conditioning and cross-training exercise for other sports, including running.

These are contrarian views, and studies to prove them would require a corporate sponsor with a vested interest in walking—like a shoe company. Bridgewater was receptive to my scientific rationale for the studies, so we shook hands, and I became the walking consultant for NaturalSport walking shoes. That handshake resulted in two landmark walking studies that clearly demonstrate that the walking gait has far greater exercise potential than the exercise community, coaches, and athletes are aware of.

WALKING INTENSITY STUDY

On December 11, 1990, a draft of the first study funded by NaturalSport was delivered to me. It was conducted at Dr. Kenneth Cooper's Institute for Aerobics Research, and it convincingly demonstrated that increased walking intensity can produce the cardiovascular fitness level and caloric expenditure of a runner without the injury associated with running.

The title of the study was "Walking for Fitness—Walking for Health: How Much Is Enough?" The study, conducted by Dr. John J. Duncan, isolated and tested the three intensity levels of exercise walking: stroll (20 minutes per mile), brisk (15 minutes per mile), and aerobic (12 minutes per mile). The study was started in September 1989 and completed in the late summer of 1990. It involved 102 premenopausal, sedentary women with an age range of 20 to 40. These women were randomly selected from the Dallas–Ft. Worth metroplex area. They all had to be nonsmokers, to consume fewer than four alcoholic drinks a day, to not be on a diet, and to be free from cardiac, pulmonary, and/or musculoskeletal disease. They also were not to have exercised more than one day a week for the previous six months. It was important to start with a group of women who were sedentary but physically well enough to complete the required walking.

At the beginning of the study, I met with all the walkers and gave them some tips on posture, stretching, and walking technique. Most of the participants were working women who wanted to break out of their sedentary rut and find an exercise they could do for a lifetime. They were eager to learn, and some of them even came at 6:00 A.M. to get their daily walks in before going to work. After thorough treadmill testing and baseline evaluation, the walkers started their supervised program. A control group was also tested and sent home to remain sedentary during the study.

The first sentence in the study stated: "Frequency, intensity, and duration provide the framework for developing an exercise prescription." In this study, frequency and duration were the same for all participants; only the walking intensity was varied. All the women walked five days a week. All groups started at 1.5 miles a day the first week, and their distances were progressively increased over the next 14 weeks until they all were walking 3.0 miles a day. This distance remained constant for the balance of the study.

The 12-minute-mile walkers were nicknamed the Green Berets because they were a tough bunch and liked the challenge of the high-intensity walk. I taught them the aerobic-walking technique that you will learn in Chapter 6, and they picked it up easily. I want to emphasize that I did not teach them race walking. They walked just like the brisk (15-minute-mile) walkers except for the bent-arm swing technique. Walking distance, duration in total time and miles, and exercise heart rate were logged daily, and were verified by a trained exercise physiologist, who supervised all sessions.

Perhaps the most interesting sidelight of the study occurred with the 20-minute-mile walkers. They started from their sedentary state fairly content with this slow pace, but in less than three months they were bored to tears. Their average age was about 30, and they were finding that it was not only boring but unchallenging to walk this slowly day after day once they attained some degree of fitness. So I got a call from Dr. Duncan. He was having a "walkers' revolt." Some of this 20-minute-mile group wanted to drop out because they didn't want to walk for three more months at this slow pace. We agreed to let the truly discontented ones increase their pace to 18 or 19 minutes per mile. Dr. Duncan held a meeting with the rebels, and, with all the southern charm and persuasion he could muster, he convinced them to continue at their slow pace.

One of the things he had to promise them, however, was that, when the study was over, I would teach them how to do the aerobic walk. Part of their discontent was in watching the aerobic walkers zip by them day after day to complete their walk in 36 minutes instead of the hour it took them. To these working women, that extra 24 minutes a day was precious time.

There is an important message for all exercise walkers in this little sidelight. Even though you may be sedentary and unfit when you start walking, in time your system will adapt to the slow, strolling pace of a 20-minute mile. You will find that a sustained slow pace is no longer challenging. All you have to do then is increase the pace of your walk enough to challenge your physiological system again. Don't make any abrupt, dramatic increase in intensity; simply pick up the pace gradually until you have a feeling of exertion during your walk and pleasant fatigue at the end.

WALKING INTENSITY MAKES A DIFFERENCE

The results of this scientifically controlled study can be used as a guide for anyone, including doctors who want to prescribe an exercise-walking program based on frequency, duration, and dose-related intensity. Over the past five years that I have been giving walking clinics, better than half the people—and sometimes 75 percent of the women—are walking for weight loss or weight maintenance. Weight is a major concern in this underexercised, overfed nation. Since exercise is recommended extensively for caloric expenditure, let's review that part of the study first.

In regard to caloric expenditure, the study said: "If the primary purpose of the exercise prescription is for weight control and body composition improvements, intensity may be an important determinant." The old saying that walking a mile burns the same amount of calories whether you walk slow or fast is finally laid to rest. The study unequivocally stated: "Contrary to popular belief, we found that walking an identical distance at a lower intensity–longer duration does not provide the same kilocaloric [kilocalories are what we all refer to as calories] energy expenditure as walking at a higher intensity for a shorter duration."

To break this statement down into meaningful numbers, the study explained: "The gross rate of energy expenditure per 3-mile workout was 53 percent *greater* in the high intensity–short duration group (12 minute/mile) compared to the combination of low intensity–long duration group (20 minute/mile), and 26 percent greater when compared to the moderate intensity–moderate duration group (15 minute/mile). . . . Walking 3 miles per day at a

12 minute/mile pace, five days per week, would expend 30,680 more kilocalories per year than would the same walking program at a 20 minute/mile pace."

The additional 30,680 calories that an aerobic walker burns walking the 12-minute-mile pace represents almost 9 pounds of weight loss. (Note: 3,500 calories = 1 pound of body weight). What's even more important is that those extra calories were burned while walking 2 hours less a week than the strollers. The 20-minute-mile walkers walked 5 hours a week to burn fewer calories than the aerobic walkers, who walked only 3 hours per week. If the slow walkers in the study had known this, then Dr. Duncan might not have been able to put down that revolt.

I mentioned earlier that this was the first study measuring the 12-minute-mile level of walking intensity among women. Supporting this study's findings, one on male college students was reported in the President's Council on Physical Fitness walking booklet. That study stated: "Walking's conditioning effects improve dramatically at speeds faster than 3 miles per hour (20-minute miles). At that rate, the college students burned an average of 66 calories per mile. When they increased their pace to 5 miles per hour (12-minute miles), they used up 124 calories per mile." You don't have to take college math to see that this is only 8 calories shy of doubling the number of calories burned. Indeed, walking intensity dramatically affects energy expenditure. It all goes back to the principle of gait efficiency.

WALKING TO THE AEROBIC FITNESS OF A RUNNER

I have referred often to the fact that walking is continually excluded from lists of exercises vigorous enough to produce a top aerobic fitness level. The evidence is now conclusive that exercise walking can be as effective as running for aerobic fitness. Like caloric expenditure, aerobic fitness or cardiorespiratory fitness is directly related to the intensity level of the walker.

The cardiovascular system governs aerobic capacity, and heart rate reflects the amount of effort expended during exercise. *Aerobic capacity* refers to the maximum rate at which one's body can use oxygen. The aerobic walkers in our study demonstrated clearly that a maximum heart rate *can* be achieved by walking. The brisk walkers (15-minute mile) also attained an elevated heart rate, and

Dr. Duncan observed, "For those who are interested in obtaining meaningful improvements in cardiorespiratory fitness, moderate to fast walking provides the necessary physiologic stimulus to accomplish this goal."

This part of the study gave me great satisfaction. I don't have a degree in exercise physiology; however, it was as obvious to me as an elephant in the pantry that if the two main objectives of exercise are to elevate the heart rate and to burn calories by using the major muscle groups in the body, the walking gait accomplishes both because it becomes highly inefficient the faster we walk. Why on earth, then, have we all been continually advised by exercise experts to shift from walking to running, which is the most *efficient* (and injurious) gait?

Apparently the answer to this question is that most of those involved with exercise physiology focus on walking and running from the perspective of speed rather than of gait efficiency. When the walking gait is elevated to a highly inefficient pace, as it was in the study, the exercise results are impressive. NaturalSport's study (see Figure 4.1) showed that the aerobic walkers (12-minute mile) exercised at an average of 86 percent (163 beats per minute) of their maximal heart rate capacity. The brisk walkers (15-minute mile) also did well. They trained at an average of 67 percent (126 beats per minute), while the strollers (20 minutes mile) trained at 56 percent (106 beats per minute) of their maximal heart rate.

Once the walkers reached their assigned walking intensity levels at the 3-mile distance, their heart rates plateaued. The strollers (20-minute mile) could have strolled for another six months and their heart rates would have remained at about 106 beats per minute. As you begin a walking program, remember that the body adjusts to the demands placed on it. An amount of exercise that elevated your heart rate to your target zone last month may not provide enough intensity to do so this month. To increase your fitness from a lower to a higher level, you have to ask your heart to work a little harder by simply walking a little faster.

This was demonstrated by our brisk walkers (15-minute mile), who reached 67 percent (126 beats per minute) of their maximal heart rate. That is a significant improvement, and it did not require any change in walking technique. Up until now, I have been comparing the fitness improvement and caloric expenditure differences between the aerobic walkers and the strollers, but it is time to give

FIGURE 4.1

Walking for fitness—walking for health: How much is enough?

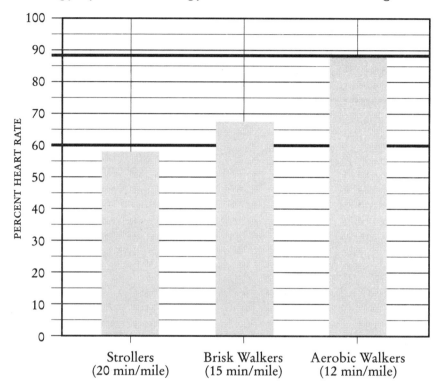

SOURCE: NaturalSport Walking Study, Institute for Aerobics Research, Dallas, Texas.

appropriate attention to the moderate-paced, brisk walkers. Their caloric expenditure of 269 was only 71 less than that of the aerobic walkers, and their heart rate indicated they were getting a good workout.

Brisk walking is a sustainable, doable pace for any healthy person who does not have a physical impairment in his or her walking gait. People well into their eighties are capable of brisk walking. The brisk pace may be the best, because it falls within the range of *all* walkers.

According to the study, the VO_2 max, which is a recognized measure of cardiovascular fitness, increased in a "dose response manner from the slower (+1.4 ml/Kg/minute) to the moderate (+3.0 ml/Kg/minute) and to the fastest (+5.0 ml/Kg/minute)." The term *ml/Kg/minute* is an abbreviation for "milliliter per kilogram per minute." That doesn't mean much to those of us who aren't exercise physiologists, but the numbers do. They indicate the level of VO_2 max improvement that these walking groups achieved from their original sedentary state and compared with the sedentary control group. The strollers (+1.4), brisk walkers (+3.0), and aerobic walkers (+5.0) all showed progressive improvement based on intensity. The study stated: "The VO_2 max differed significantly between the 12 minute/mile and the sedentary control group and the 15 minute/mile and control group, but contrasts between the 20 minute/mile and control group were not significantly different."

The slow stroll is the safe pace for everyone to begin a walking program, but, as the study indicated, if you never progress beyond it, you will not improve your cardiorespiratory capacity significantly. The reason is that the 20-minute-mile stroll is also the most energy-efficient pace within the human walking gait. It puts the least demand for oxygen on the cardiorespiratory system; consequently, it provides very little improvement of VO_2 max over the sedentary state. According to Professor Taylor's research on animal locomotion, animals usually select "an energetically optimal speed for each gait." It appears that a 20-minute-mile stroll is close to the energetically optimal speed for the human walking gait.

The number that was of great interest to me, and one of the main reasons for conducting this study, was the VO_2 max improvement for the aerobic walkers. I was curious about how their improvement (+5.0 ml/Kg/min), would compare with that of people who run for exercise. Dr. Duncan said, "There have been numerous VO_2 max tests on runners, and the 5-milliliter improvement for our 12-minute-mile walkers would compare favorably to that of an average exercise runner." Figure 4.2, a chart constructed by Dr. Duncan, shows the percentage of cardiorespiratory improvement at the different walking intensity levels. Note that the aerobic walker's results equal those of a runner. The study results coincide with my own and my wife's treadmill fitness test results at the Cooper Clinic. We also have the fitness levels of runners from our aerobic walking.

In addition to increased cardiorespiratory fitness, there was an

FIGURE 4.2

Walking for fitness—walking for health: How much is enough?

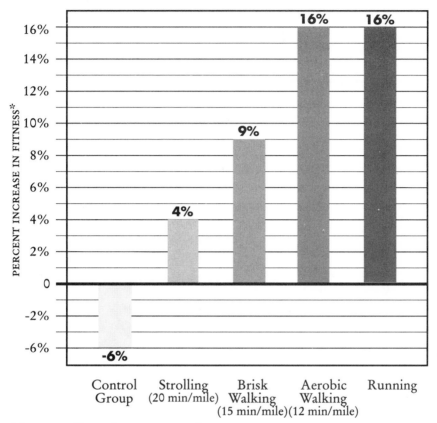

*As measured by maximum oxygen uptake

SOURCE: NaturalSport Walking Study, Institute for Aerobics Research, Dallas, Texas.

increase in HDL (the good cholesterol) that amounted to a 12 to 18 percent reduction in the risk of coronary disease among all the walkers, regardless of walking intensity. The strollers did as well as the aerobic walkers, but it took them 2 hours longer each week to achieve the same results.

During the study, the three groups walked an accumulated total in excess of 20,000 miles. As the study stated, "Unlike most other

modes of exercise, walking at higher intensities did not come at
the expense of a greater risk of orthopedic injury." The study
noted, "None of the women in the 12, 15, or 20 minute/mile groups
sustained a walking related injury which necessitated consultation
with a physician. . . . Thus, moderate-to-fast walking provides a
safe and effective means for women to achieve significant gains in
cardiorespiratory fitness." I've said it already in this book, and I
say it at all my walking clinics: the only thing running will give
you that walking won't is *injury*!

The proper prescription for exercise depends on the needs, goals,
and abilities of each participant. The walking study provides a
sliding scale of intensity and amount of time necessary to increase
cardiorespiratory fitness, cardiovascular health, or both. The study
concluded: "For those interested in exercising for cardiorespiratory
fitness or weight control, desired responses are achieved in a dose
dependent gradient, with walking at higher intensities producing
the greatest gains." As mentioned in Chapter 1, there is a distinct
difference between health and fitness. You can be highly fit and
terribly unhealthy. For those interested in cardiovascular health,
walking frequently and with adequate duration, regardless of intensity, is extremely beneficial.

Finally, the study recommended: *"Emphasis should be placed
on factors that result in permanent behavioral lifestyle changes while
encouraging the pursuit of a lifetime of activity"* (emphasis in original). I promised Dr. Duncan that I would make sure everybody
got this message. It all boils down to this: if you take up a physical
activity like exercise walking for the rest of your life, with enough
frequency and duration and at whatever intensity you will do it
consistently, you'll make a major contribution to your health, longevity, and quality of life. All it costs you is a little time.

LEVELS OF WALKING INTENSITY

I believe the term *exercise walking* is the most appropriate umbrella
under which the various levels of walking intensity can be artic-
ulated. Two terms currently used for walking are *fitness walking*
and *health walking*. These are generic terms, but they are not
quantifiable in relation to exercise intensity. *Fitness walking* has a
nice ring to it, but we don't say fitness cycling, fitness swimming,
or fitness running. People say that they cycle, swim, or run. It

should be noted that *exercise* was specifically defined in the CDC Workshop as "planned, structured, and repetitive bodily movement." Thus, it follows that *exercise walking* denotes a structured physical movement, as opposed to walking that is part of normal daily activities.

Walking has four quantifiable intensity levels, and I will give them to you in minutes per mile. All too often walking pace is referred to in miles per hour, such as 3 or 4 miles per hour. Some people don't know how to convert miles per hour to minutes per mile; besides, runners never refer to their speed in miles per hour. A runner will say, "I run 10-minute miles," not 6 miles per hour. We walkers must get rid of that old slowpoke designation also. We can get just as fit as runners.

Here are the four measurable intensity levels for exercising walking in terms of minutes per mile:

STROLLING—*Low Intensity. To stroll* is a term familiar to everyone. It is defined in the dictionary as "to walk leisurely as inclination directs." Strolling constitutes most of our normal daily walking. It starts as slow as 30 minutes per mile and increases to about 18 minutes per mile at the top end of its range. Part of the definition, "as inclination directs," accurately describes how people arrive at their normal walking pace in the course of their daily activities.

Within the 30-minute- to 18-minute-mile range, most walkers will find a comfortable, energy-efficient pace that suits their needs. The next time you are walking somewhere that doesn't require haste, check what kind of strolling groove you are in. The average person will comfortably stroll along at about 20 to 24 minutes per mile.

Strolling is the pace recommended for most people who are starting an exercise-walking program from a sedentary state. It is particularly recommended for the obese, cardiac rehabilitation patients, and the elderly. At the Cooper Wellness Program, where I conduct monthly walking clinics, we may have all three of these types in one class.

Some obese participants find it is a struggle merely to walk at the slow end of the strolling range, even for short distances. People who are obese frequently have high blood pressure and are in a life-threatening condition. Happily, I have observed some re-

long-term success stories in conquering obesity—stories
:d with that first tentative strolling step on an exercise-
........g program.

BRISK WALKING—*Moderate Intensity. Brisk* is also a term familiar
to most people, and it is used frequently to designate an accelerated
walking pace. In the dictionary it is defined as "quick and active;
lively: a brisk walk." The brisk pace starts at about 17 minutes per
mile pace at the slow end of the range and tops out at 14 minutes
per mile. Most fit walkers handle a 15-minute-mile pace comfortably.

Brisk walking is within the range of any healthy individual, but
it is not the pace at which you should begin a walking program
unless you are already reasonably fit. The walking booklet from
the President's Council on Physical Fitness states, "Eventually,
your goal should be to get to the place where you can comfortably
walk 3 miles in 45 minutes. . . . We recommend that you walk as
briskly as your condition permits."

In the August 1988 issue of *The Physician and Sportsmedicine*,
Barry Franklin, Ph.D., director of the Cardiac Rehabilitation and
Exercise Laboratories at William Beaumont Hospital in Royal
Oak, Michigan, and a member of the magazine's editorial board,
said, "For the average person, walking may be the best method of
becoming fit. Eight of ten people will improve their fitness with
regular, brisk walking."

AEROBIC WALKING—*High Intensity. Aerobic walking* is not a
term familiar to most exercisers, but it ranges from about a 13.5-
minute-mile pace at the low end up to a 10.0-minute-mile pace at
the fast end. In this range, the two human gaits—walking and
running—overlap. This fast-walking pace is in the same range that
a slow run or jog begins. Most fit walkers who learn aerobic walking generally level off at about 12.0 to 12.5 minutes per mile.

If you are a formerly sedentary person who has begun walking
and you progress in fitness from a stroll to brisk walking, your
heart rate will plateau below your aerobic-training range unless
you increase your walking pace. If you want to increase your
cardiovascular fitness level and burn more calories for weight control, you will have to put more intensity into your walk in order
to elevate your heart rate. The aerobic-walking technique in Chap-

ter 6 will teach you how to achieve this intensity in the walking gait without having to switch to another aerobic exercise.

Confusion over what to call fast exercise walking occurs at the highest levels. In the July 1990 issue of *The Physician and Sportsmedicine*, in an article entitled "President Bush: He's Busy, but He Still Makes Time for Exercise," Dr. Burton J. Lee III (the physician to the president) revealed some of President Bush's exercise routines. Dr. Lee mentioned that at Camp David on weekends the president "sometimes conducts 'power walks.' " When the interviewer asked, "What are power walks?" Dr. Lee replied, "He just walks so darn fast that everybody disappears." That's hardly a usable definition of walking intensity, and I suspect that President Bush, who is primarily a runner, is merely the best of a bunch of slow walkers. I would bet my quail dog that he couldn't outwalk my wife, Carol.

I named my first book *Aerobic Walking* because it dealt with this walking intensity and the benefits derived from it. Terms such as *power walking, speedwalking, pacewalking*, and *health walking* are simply not quantifiable. One person's fitness may be another's unfitness. Speedwalking for some may only be brisk walking for others. By contrast, the aerobic intensity is quantifiable. If you are walking and your heart rate is in your aerobic training range, then you are aerobic walking.

RACE WALKING—*Very High Intensity.* Race walking is a judged track and field event and has been part of the Olympic Summer Games since 1908. Currently there are two races for men—20K (12.4 miles) and 50K (31.1 miles). In the 1992 Olympics, a women's 10K (6.2 miles) race will be added. Unless you are in a slow field of older walkers, race walking starts at about a 10-minute-mile-pace. As of this writing, the male world record for the mile is 5:33.50, held by an American, Tim Lewis. The female record is 6:16.72, held by Sada Eidikite of the Soviet Union. Most people can't even run that fast flat out. These race-walking records are remarkable athletic achievements.

I consider race walking a competitive sport and not a daily exercise. In Chapter 9, I cover the rules of race walking and the technique necessary to become a competitive walker. When people start walking beyond the top range of the brisk pace, especially if they have their arms bent and pumping vigorously, there is a tendency to classify that as race walking. Believe me, it is not; it is simply walking in the extended-gait range that is aerobic walking.

ESTABLISHING YOUR FREQUENCY, DURATION, AND INTENSITY

The NaturalSport walking study was conducted in a controlled environment with daily supervision. Each participant had been given a thorough physical and treadmill test. The frequency, duration, and intensity of the walkers were preset. Not much could go wrong physically with the participants, and it didn't. If you walk five days a week, 3 miles per day, and select one of the intensity levels (20, 15, or 12 minutes per mile), you can expect results similar to those of the study participants, whether you are male or female.

Not everybody can walk five days a week, however; others may be able to walk more. Is 3 miles the right distance for everybody? If not, how much is? The walkers in the study all started at 1.5 miles. Should everybody start at that distance? Once you have achieved a good fitness level, how much walking is necessary to maintain it? These questions should be answered and your initial fitness level established *before* you start exercise walking.

This book will be read by people with a wide range of fitness levels—or, more probably, *unfitness* levels. I won't be able to observe your tolerance for exercise, so I will assume that everyone is starting from sedentary. Many people get turned off by exercise when they rush into it from a sedentary state without regard for their physical tolerance. A number of things can happen—most of them bad. Above all, don't start exercising with the expectation that you will immediately experience some feeling of exhilaration and sense of well-being. Those will come later.

When approaching any kind of exercise, it is always best to err on the conservative side. To establish your initial fitness level, approach it like putting your toe in the bathwater to check the temperature—very slowly and carefully. Finding out that you are capable of doing more is a pleasant surprise. Finding out that you did too much too soon is a pain in the buns—literally. The beauty of exercise walking is that there is no reason for you ever to experience soreness or discomfort.

The scientific way to establish a fitness level would be a treadmill stress test. If your doctor thinks you should have one, I recommend you follow his advice. He may have good reason. However, for the average person who is starting an exercise-walking program, that is not necessary. All you need to do is take your first walk at a controlled, comfortable pace.

I recommend that you measure your walking fitness level in terms of miles instead of minutes. For instance, measure out a 1-, 2-, or 3-mile course in your neighborhood with your car odometer. Make a mental note of where the ½-mile marks are. That way you will know approximately how far you walked the first time. Was it ½ mile, 1 mile, or longer? How far you went is more important than how long it took. Don't try for a fast pace. Whatever distance you covered becomes your fitness baseline. From that distance you will slowly add on the miles. Intensity comes much later.

In some big cities, where people walk in parks (like Central Park in New York City), or in shopping malls, it is not easy to get exact distances. In that case, measure your first walk by how many minutes it took. If you walked 18 minutes, for example, without any discomfort, then your fitness baseline will increase from the 18-minute level. Whether you measure in minutes or miles, do not walk to the point of exhaustion. Always quit while you have a little energy left.

In establishing a fitness level, I favor measuring the walk by distance because, as you progress, your fitness level will increase and so will your pace. The combination of distance and time is the best way to track your intensity level. An easy way to measure your progress is to check your time against a chosen distance. For instance, you may want to know how long it takes for you to walk 3 miles this month, then see if you can walk it even faster next month.

Frequency: How Often Should You Walk?

Is it better to walk 90 minutes one day a week or 30 minutes a day three days a week? In my walking clinics, the question of how many days a week to walk comes up often. People who have the time and who thoroughly enjoy their walks should walk every day, or as many days as possible. As was established in the walking study—and in the 3 million years since Lucy—frequency does not cause injury.

Exercise walking should become your foundation exercise for a lifetime. Approach it on the basis not of how little you can get by with but of how often and how much you can do. I can't emphasize strongly enough that if you are trying to lose weight you should walk seven days a week. Each minute and each mile that you walk you are doing the best exercise possible for weight loss.

However, not everybody can walk every day, so the question is, How many days does it take to get some positive exercise results? I have found the widely used college textbook *Exercise Physiology: Energy, Nutrition, and Human Performance* by William D. McArdle, Frank I. Katch, and Victor L. Katch an excellent source to answer questions like this. I will be quoting from it from time to time, so at this point it seems simpler to reduce its long title to *Exercise Physiology*.

In answer to the foregoing question, *Exercise Physiology* states, "Fewer than two days a week generally does not produce adequate changes in either anaerobic or aerobic capacity or body composition." We are not concerned with anaerobic capacity, but we are with the other two. In a summary of six studies that investigated optimal exercise frequency for weight reduction, the textbook says, "It was observed that training 2 days a week did not change body weight, fat folds, or percent body fat. Training 3 and 4 days a week, however, had a significant effect. . . . Subjects who trained 4 days a week reduced their body weight and fat folds significantly more than the 3 days per week group." Now you know why I said walking seven days a week should be the goal for anyone in a serious weight-loss program.

Other than for weight loss, the required frequency of exercise walking depends on the level of fitness you desire and the intensity you are willing to put into it. For instance, if you intend to walk at less than the brisk 15-minute-mile pace, you probably should walk five or six days a week. While this will give you only a low to moderate level of fitness, it will still benefit your overall health. Any exercise that contributes to your health is worthwhile. Don't become preoccupied with fitness only.

Duration: How Long Should You Walk?

I have found that most people who become avid exercise walkers end up averaging about 3 miles per walk. Time permitting, and especially on weekends, they tend to walk farther. My daily walk is usually 5 miles, whether I go slow, moderate, or fast. I rarely go slow, because this is my individual preference, but that doesn't mean you shouldn't walk at a slower pace. I am retired, so I have the time to walk 5 miles every day. This exercise time is as important a part of my daily routine as bathing or brushing my teeth. Unfortunately, there are millions of retired people in this country who don't walk at all. Walking even 1 mile would be a worthwhile contribution to their health.

Three miles per walk is a good exercise goal, and it is consistent with the recommendation of the President's Council on Physical Fitness. However, *Exercise Physiology* points out that "a threshold duration per workout has *not* been identified for optimal cardiovascular improvement" (emphasis in original). It concludes: "Such a threshold is probably dependent on many factors including the total work done, exercise intensity, training frequency, and initial fitness level." The variables of frequency, duration, and intensity are inextricably linked and can be manipulated to produce varying exercise results.

Intensity: How Fast Should You Walk To Attain and Maintain Fitness?

On the relationship of duration and intensity of exercise, *Exercise Physiology* states: "With high-intensity training, significant improvements occur with 10 to 15 minute exercise periods per workout. Conversely, a 45 minute continuous exercise period may be required to produce a training effect when exercise intensity is below the threshold heart rate." The textbook concludes: "*It appears that the lower intensity of exercise is offset by the increased duration of training*" (emphasis in original). Simply stated, if you are going to walk with less intensity, you should plan on walking for a longer duration.

Exercise intensity is essential in attaining fitness, especially aerobic fitness. Just as important, it is critical in *maintaining* fitness. Often in the question-and-answer part of my walking clinics, the question comes up, "Will I have to walk every day for the rest of my life to stay fit?" It takes persistence and the right combination of frequency, duration, and intensity to move a normal, healthy person from a sedentary state to an elevated level of aerobic fitness. Maintaining that level, however, can be accomplished with less frequency and duration than were needed to achieve it—as long as the intensity is maintained.

In a study cited in *Exercise Physiology*, healthy young adults using a combination of cycling and running 40 minutes a day for six days a week over a 10-week period achieved a 25 percent improvement in VO$_2$ max. They were then split into two groups, one of which reduced exercise frequency to four days a week and the other to two days a week. However, both groups exercised for an additional 15 weeks at the same intensity and duration. In both groups the gains in aerobic capacity were maintained.

The same exercise model was used to study the effects of reduced training duration on the maintenance of aerobic fitness. Following the initial 10-week protocol of the other exercisers, these participants continued the same intensity and frequency of training for an additional 15 weeks, but they reduced training duration from the original 40 minutes to 26 or 13 minutes per day. *Exercise Physiology* reports, "Despite this reduction in training duration by as much as two-thirds almost all of the VO$_2$ max and performance increases were maintained."

The only other variable to manipulate in exercise maintenance is the intensity of exercise. On this aspect, *Exercise Physiology* says: "When the intensity of training is reduced and the frequency and duration held constant even a one-third reduction in work rate causes the VO$_2$ max to *decline. . . . If exercise intensity is maintained, the frequency and duration of physical activity required to maintain a certain level of aerobic fitness is less than that required to improve it*" (emphasis in original). The textbook concludes: "This strongly suggests that training intensity plays a principal role in maintaining the increase in aerobic power achieved through training." The term *training* in this instance is used in place of *exercise*.

The foregoing is extremely useful information for every exerciser, particularly for people who say they don't have time to exercise regularly and as a result don't exercise at all. I find that most people believe that once they start an exercise program they have to keep up the same regimen every day or they will lose fitness. This assumption discourages some people from making an exercise commitment. As the studies just cited show, this is not the case.

Exercise walkers have great flexibility in maintaining their fitness levels by simply keeping up their intensity of exercise while reducing frequency or duration. The study cited in *Exercise Physi-*

ology clearly shows that an exerciser can reduce frequency by as much as half and still maintain aerobic fitness. Getting an elevated aerobic-fitness level still requires the initial commitment of three or four months. Thereafter, however, a lifetime of fitness can be maintained with more flexibility and in less time than most people realize.

How Quickly is Fitness Lost?

Another question that comes up frequently is "If I have to quit exercising for a while for health or other reasons, how quickly do I lose my fitness?" When exercising stops, *Exercise Physiology* says, a significant decline in aerobic capacity occurs within two weeks. It further states: "After 12 weeks almost all of the training adaptations [i.e., improvements] return to pre-training levels." It doesn't take long to go from fit back to sedentary. The old saying "Use it or lose it" certainly applies to exercise.

The Aerobic Training Range

Adding intensity to an exercise regimen elevates the heart rate, and, if enough intensity is added and maintained for 20 minutes or longer, an "aerobic-training effect" is achieved. There are several ways to monitor the heart rate's response to increased exercise intensity, but the formula most widely used by exercisers and athletes is the one in the American College of Sports Medicine *Guidelines for Exercise Testing and Prescription*. It is "Predicted maximal heart rate (MHR) = 220 − age." The guidelines state: "Considerable variability ($+/-$ 15 beats min^{-1}) is associated with this estimate of maximal heart rate."

Using this equation, an aerobic training range of 65 to 85 percent of maximal heart rate for a 40-year-old would be 220 − 40 = 180; .65 × 180 = 117 and .85 × 180 = 153. Thus, a 40-year-old's aerobic-training range measured by heart rate would be 117 to 153. The guidelines caution: "The target heart rate range is only a *guideline* to follow in prescribing exercise" (emphasis in original). They add that judgment must be used about how an individual responds to exercise. If necessary, the intensity should be altered to provide comfort and safety while you are trying to achieve a training effect. Using this equation, Table 4.1 lists the 65 to 85 percent training range for ages 20 through 80.

TABLE 4.1.

Aerobic training range (65 to 85 percent of maximum heart rate)

AGE	20	25	30	35	40	45	50	55	60	65	70	75	80
65%	130	126	123	120	117	113	110	107	104	100	97	94	91
85%	170	166	161	157	153	149	144	140	136	132	128	123	119

A word of caution: Certain medicines, such as beta blockers, alter the heart rate. Consult with your physician about what your exercising heart rate should be if you are on any type of prescription medication.

WALKING GUIDELINES

Using the frequency, duration, and intensity components of exercise, we can create some general exercise-walking guidelines in terms of how often, how far, and how fast. I emphasize that these are guidelines *only*. A walking program should ultimately match the fitness level, time constraints, and physical limitations of the individual walker and his or her personal exercise goals. One thing I am absolutely unwavering about, however: you should always achieve your frequency and duration goals before you attempt intensity.

How Often: Four days a week minimum, up to seven days a week for those trying to lose weight. Unlike runners, walkers do not incur injury from frequency of exercise.

How Far: Walk as far as possible without undue stress to establish your personal-fitness baseline. Gradually increase that distance to 3 miles, but do not increase it at a rate of more than ¼ mile every three or four days, or a total of ½ mile per week. Almost everyone except the extremely obese can handle this amount without soreness or unnecessary fatigue. I know many can do more, but it is better to err on the conservative side. If you are trying to lose weight, extend your walk as far beyond 3 miles as time permits.

How Fast: For aerobic fitness, walk at an intensity that will put your heart rate into the 65 to 85 percent aerobic-training range. In achieving your walking intensity, remember that your *heart rate is always more important than minutes per mile*. A high heart rate at a relatively slow pace means that you are not fit enough to go faster safely. As your fitness level rises, your heart rate will drop; then you can gradually increase your pace. For a moderate fitness level, use the brisk 15-minute-mile pace.

A Good Rule of Thumb: Walk at least four days a week, and walk as far and as fast as it takes to achieve your personal exercise goals.

5

STRETCHING, POSTURE, STROLLING, AND BRISK WALKING

STRETCHING AND FLEXIBILITY

I have conducted numerous walking clinics for several thousand people, and I can say with accuracy that less than 20 percent of exercise walkers do any stretching of their walking muscles. Those who do some stretching generally are the faster-paced walkers or race walkers.

Addressing the importance of stretching and flexibility, Mayo Clinic physical therapist Phil Orte explained in the October 1990 issue of the clinic's monthly health letter that flexibility is one of the "three pillars of fitness," along with muscular strength and cardiovascular endurance. "Flexibility is important for daily life as well as athletics," Orte observed. "Getting older doesn't automatically mean getting stiffer. Careful stretching can help you stay flexible."

Mayo Clinic physicians and physical therapists recommend stretching as an integral part of all exercise. They say: "Stretching can help you: (1) Increase the amount of stress (such as bearing weight or enduring repeated movement) that your muscles and tendons can withstand. (2) Maintain joint and muscle flexibility.

(3) Maintain or improve a range of motion that the particular activity you choose doesn't offer."

Flexibility is the ability of the joints to move through their full range of motion, and for the muscles to approach their maximum stretchability. Flexibility will vary from joint to joint and person to person. Don't be alarmed if you can't attain the same flexibility in a joint or stretch in a muscle that your walking partner can. Simply work on getting the maximum flexibility possible for you. An exercise walker uses all the major muscle groups in the lower body; stretching these muscles and having the joints they influence flexible are important for a fluid, rhythmic walk.

The type of stretching you should do is called *static stretching*, which simply means that you stretch the muscle slowly to its greatest possible length and hold it for a specified time. Then slowly release the tension on the muscle. Stretch until you feel a pulling sensation, with a slight bit of discomfort or a minor, dull ache. You should not feel pain, and above all you should not bounce or snap the muscle. Over time, stretching will produce a semi-permanent lengthening of the muscle. It is semipermanent because if you stop doing it the muscle will shorten again, in time, especially if you are older.

There are many ways to stretch the same muscle or muscle group. I have chosen the exercises that I think are the easiest to adapt to almost any situation. A great many stretches require being on the ground or on the floor. I have eliminated those because, if walking outdoors or in a shopping mall, most people would not want to get down on the ground.

Dr. Dennis Humphrey of the Biomedical Sciences Department at Southwest Missouri State University, who often writes the "Exercise Adviser" column for *The Physician and Sportsmedicine*, suggested a series of easy stretches with simple instructions. He says, "The proper way to stretch is to first warm-up with brisk walking for 2–5 minutes." It is best to warm up with the type of exercise you are going to do. Runners jog and walkers walk. Warm muscles are more elastic, and their stretching is more effective.

If you are just starting a stretching and flexibility program, Dr. Humphrey advises, "Repeat each stretching exercise five times and hold the stretch for a count of 10. As your flexibility increases you may hold the stretch for a count of 20 to 30 and you may repeat the stretch up to 10 times. Remember to breathe regularly." Like all exercises, stretching takes more effort and frequency to improve from zero to a desirable level than it does to maintain that level. For example, Dr. Humphrey says, "You should perform the stretching exercises 3 to 5 days per week to *increase* flexibility, but you only need to do them 2 to 3 days per week to *maintain* flexibility. More than 5 days per week is not necessary."

I am going to give you three priority stretches that I guarantee will help you walk better. These involve the muscles or muscle groups that contribute to the walking gait. Obviously, we should do more stretches from an overall flexibility standpoint, but this chapter is concerned only with getting your walking program started.

The muscle groups that contribute most to the walking gait are (1) hamstrings (back of the thighs); (2) calf muscles; and (3) quadriceps (front of the thighs). It is a close call whether the calf muscles are more important than the hamstrings. Race-walking coaches will argue that they are. From a pure propulsion standpoint, that may be true, but I have found that more people (especially older people) need to work more on their shortened hamstrings than on their calf muscles, so we will start with them.

Hamstrings Stretch

If you recall Chapter 2, the main function of the hamstrings is to decelerate and stop the leg on the forward swing so the walker can plant his or her heel. The hamstrings are attached to both the back of the knee and the pelvis, so they also flex the knee at toe-off as the leg starts its forward swing, lifting the foot and permitting the toes to clear the ground as they pass under the body. Shortened hamstrings cause shortened stride lengths. At the end of the forward leg swing, if your hamstrings cannot reach their full extension, the heel of your front foot will land at a shorter distance from your back foot than it normally would. You will have a short, choppy stride.

There are at least eight ways to stretch the hamstrings, but one Dr. Humphrey used in his "Exercise Adviser" column (see Figure 5.1) seems to be the simplest and most adaptable to various exercise situations. I particularly like it because it doesn't require extensive bending of the back or getting on the floor. I have one of those backs that doesn't straighten up every time I bend over.

Stand with one foot on a bench or chair, with the toes of the

FIGURE 5.1   **FIGURE 5.2**

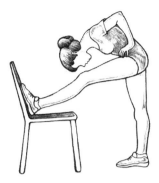

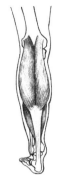

elevated foot pointing straight up. Make sure both legs are straight and the knees locked. There is a tendency to bend the knee of the weight-bearing leg, but keep it straight at all times. Place your hands on your hips and *slowly* bend forward, trying to touch your nose to the knee of your raised leg. You will immediately feel the tension in the hamstring muscles in your raised leg. *Don't bounce.* After the count of 10, straighten up slowly and reverse legs.

Calf Muscles and Tendon Stretch

The calf muscles supply the main propulsion of the walking gait. They are no strangers to most people because at one time or another we have all had cramps in them. Sometimes getting the toes of a foot extended under the covers in bed at night can cause the calf to knot up and make you think a pit bull has you by the leg. Because of their importance, it is worthwhile to see the calf muscles in an anatomical illustration (Figure 5.2).

The upper calf muscles are called the *gastrocnemius*; the lower calf muscles are the *soleus*. As a group, these muscles are called the *triceps surae*. The Achilles tendon hooks the calf muscles to the heel. As your weight-bearing foot passes under your body and becomes the trailing limb, your heel rises and your forefoot pushes against the ground toward toe-off. This is accomplished by a short, powerful contraction of the calf muscles.

You can readily see why having these muscles functioning at their maximum potential will contribute to your walking propul-

FIGURE 5.3   **FIGURE 5.4**

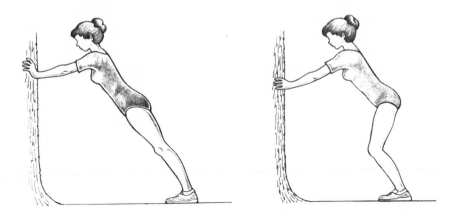

sion. The stretch I am going to give you is one used by my friend Gary Westerfield, who is a race-walking coach for some of our national champion women walkers.

Upper Calf Muscles Stretch

Stand with your feet about 18 inches apart and 3 or 4 feet from a wall (or tree, if you are outside). As in Figure 5.3, lean forward with your back straight and place both hands on the tree. Now slowly bring your hips forward while keeping your legs straight and your *heels flat on the floor*. There is a natural tendency for the heels to rise. Keep them down, however, and you will feel the pull on the *upper* calf muscles in both legs. Hold this position for the count of 10 (for beginners); then ease back with your hips.

Lower Calf Muscles and Achilles Tendon Stretch

As in Figure 5.4, with your feet, hands, and body in the same position as in the previous stretch, slowly bend your knees as if you were going to squat, but be sure to keep your heels flat on the floor. You will feel the pull on the *lower* calf muscles and Achilles tendons. Hold for the appropriate count; then slowly rise. Alternate this lower stretch with the upper stretch for the appropriate number of repetitions.

FIGURE 5.5

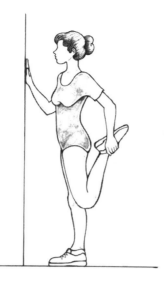

Quadriceps Stretch

The quads, as the big muscle group on the front of the thighs are commonly called, straighten the knee as your swing leg comes forward just before you plant your heel. They are connected to the patellar tendon, which goes down over the kneecap and attaches to the front of the upper part of the lower leg.

When you make your hamstrings flex your knee by pulling the lower leg up, the quads are the muscles that pull on the front of the lower leg to extend your knee and straighten the leg. The quads get their biggest workout when you are walking up a hill or up stairs. They lift your body as they straighten the knee.

Stand next to a wall or tree for balance. As in Figure 5.5, reach back and slowly pull your non-weight-bearing foot up toward your buttocks until you feel the tension or a minor, dull ache in the front thigh muscles. Don't pull the foot up sharply. Hold that for the appropriate count; then reverse legs. You should ultimately be able to touch your heels to your buttocks.

People with knee problems may not be able to get a full quad stretch, however. I fall into that category. I can get a full stretch on the left leg and only a partial stretch on the right because of my bad knee. If you have knee problems, do the best you can and take what you can get.

There is no question that if you do these three stretches you will

FIGURE 5.6   **FIGURE 5.7**

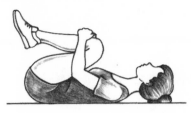
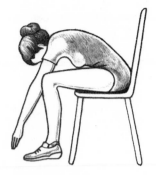

get more out of your exercise walk and will function better in your normal daily walking. I can't emphasize strongly enough that the older you get, the more important stretching and flexibility become.

There are two other stretches that I recommend you do each day after your walk. These stretches are not directly related to the propulsion of your walking gait, but they give you flexibility in an important area—the lower and middle back. Anyone who has had pain in the lower back knows the meaning of misery. Even a cough or a sneeze can make you think you are coming unhinged. These two stretches were also recommended by Dr. Humphrey. They are easy and effective.

Hip and Trunk Flexion

Lie on your back and grasp your knees (see Figure 5.6). Contract the abdominal muscles and pull your knees to your chest while pressing your lower back to the floor. If you have knee problems, pull from behind the knee at the lower end of your upper leg. Hold this position for the appropriate count; then relax a moment and repeat. Do this stretch several times a week.

Middle- and Lower-Back Stretch

Sit on a firm chair, like a kitchen chair, and spread your knees. As in Figure 5.7, slowly bend forward, with your arms outstretched and your hands together. Reach for the floor and as far forward as possible with your hands and hold for the appropriate count as you feel the pull in the lower and middle back. Do this stretch several times a week also. Those who have a potbelly will find they can't get very far down on this one. Keep trying anyhow! We'll work on that potbelly in a later chapter.

When to Stretch

According to Dr. Humphrey and every other authority on stretching, the proper procedure is
1. Warm up.
2. Do your stretching routine.
3. Engage in your exercise or sport.
4. Stretch again when you are finished and the muscles are still warm.
Now let's talk about the real world. Eighty percent of the population doesn't exercise at all. Of those who are currently exercise walking, less than 20 percent are doing any stretching.

I have found that walking a few minutes to warm up, then stopping to stretch, and then continuing my full walk is something I just don't do regularly. Here's my routine; while it is not absolutely proper, it works. I do an easy 10-count stretch of three repetitions on each of the three primary muscle groups without a warm-up. It isn't as effective without the warm-up, but it helps some. I then take my exercise walk and really get into the stretches after the walk, while my muscles are still warm. Getting the muscles stretched thoroughly at the end of your walk has the residual effect you want.

Upper-Body Stretches

Up until now, I have concentrated only on the muscles of the lower body. As you become an accomplished walker and start to pick up the pace, your upper body and arm swing will be increasingly important. You will need flexibility and looseness, particularly around the shoulder joints. This can be accomplished in the first 2 or 3 minutes of your walk.

As you begin your walk, loosen your arms and shoulders by swinging your arms across your body as if you were trying to wrap each one around your opposite side. Swing them with the right arm crossing over the left, then the left over the right. Swing them behind your back so that the fingers of the opposite hands touch. You will feel your back and shoulders loosen up after a few swings.

As you continue to walk, swing your arms around like windmills a few times, clockwise and counterclockwise. Nice, easy swings will loosen up the shoulder joints for a freer arm swing during your walk. Roll your head around clockwise and counterclockwise several times to loosen up your neck muscles. All of this can be done simultaneously with walking and warming up your leg muscles.

POSTURE, POSTURE, POSTURE

For exercise walkers, proper posture is absolutely, positively, unequivocally, without a doubt the most critical, fundamental aspect of the walk. I can't say it with any more emphasis than that! Getting the body lined up properly before you take the first step and keeping it lined up through your entire walk will give you a more rewarding, less fatiguing workout. It will also help you improve your posture during your normal daily activities.

Why is correct posture so important? The American Physical Therapy Association has the best answer: "Good posture is important because it helps your body function at top speed. It promotes movement efficiency and endurance and contributes to an over-all feeling of well being." I can transfer all those words to walkers. I have observed that the slowest walkers (strollers) generally have the poorest posture, and the fastest walkers (race walkers) have flawless posture.

Many strollers tend to walk with their heads tilted forward, their shoulders slumped, and their stomachs sagging. Don't take my word for it; start your own observation study of walkers' posture in relationship to their speed. You will find, as I did, that, as the pace of the walk picks up, the requirement for good posture increases. Brisk walkers tend to have better posture than strollers. Aerobic walkers who are reaching for the 12-minute-mile pace just can't get there without good posture. Race walkers, who require absolute "top speed" and "movement efficiency," walk with perfect posture. I have watched champion American race walkers Lynn Weik, Tim Lewis, Viisha Sedlak, Debbie Lawrence, and others compete. One thing they all have in common is perfect posture. They couldn't set records without it.

FIGURE 5.8   FIGURE 5.9

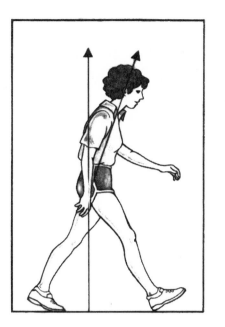

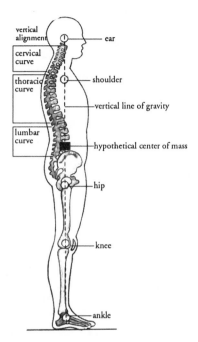

I realize that you are not taking up exercise walking to set records but to improve your fitness and quality of life. According to the American Physical Therapy Association, "Good posture is also good prevention. . . . If you have poor posture, your bones are not properly aligned and your muscles, joints, and ligaments take more strain than nature intended. Faulty posture may cause you fatigue, muscular strain, and in later stages, pain."

One of the areas of discomfort when walking with bad posture is the lower back. Lower-back pain rears its ugly head quickest for walkers with improper posture who are trying to increase their speed. When I have walkers in a clinic tell me they get a pain in the lower back when walking at a fast pace, I ask them to show me how they walk. Almost without exception they walk with the posture shown in Figure 5.8. Notice the vertical line of gravity and how the upper body is out in front of that line. The walker is increasing speed by literally falling forward. The walker releases good toning tension on the lower abdominal muscles and transfers it to the lower-back muscles, where it shouldn't be. The back muscles have to work harder to hold the torso forward of the vertical line of gravity. Unnecessary fatigue ultimately becomes discomfort and pain in the lower back.

Let's get you properly lined up before you start your walking program. The alignment shown in Figure 5.9 is the one I use in my clinics, and it is recommended by the American Physical Therapy Association.

First, notice the vertical line of gravity. This imaginary line connects the ear, shoulder, hip, knee, and ankle. It also passes through the hypothetical center of mass (black square), which I added to the figure. In Figure 5.8 the head and entire upper body were tilted in front of the vertical line of gravity, causing the body to lurch forward by the pull of gravity instead of being powered forward by the big muscle groups in the legs.

Observe the spinal column in Figure 5.9. A properly aligned, healthy back has three natural curves: a slight forward curve in the neck (cervical curve), a slight backward curve in the upper back (thoracic curve), and a slight forward curve in the lower back (lumbar curve). The American Physical Therapy Association says, "Good posture actually means keeping these three curves in balanced alignment."

Putting the body in alignment is easy, but keeping it there is not, particularly if you aren't in shape or are carrying too much weight. The muscles and joints are responsible for maintaining good posture. According to the American Physical Therapy Association, "Strong, flexible muscles are essential to good posture. Abdominal, hip, and leg muscles that are weak and inflexible cannot support your back's natural curves."

Your back's natural curves are balanced by your hip, knee, and ankle joints when you move about. Holding all of that in proper alignment while walking at a fast pace requires practice and perseverance, especially if you have had bad posture for most of your life. I had a terrible time getting my posture together, and I confess that even today on a real fast walk I'll occasionally experience fatigue and discomfort in my lower back. I check my posture, and, sure enough, I am usually leaning forward a bit. It doesn't take much, and, when I straighten up, the discomfort goes away.

The way I teach posture is to start from the head and go down, following the vertical line of gravity. Line yourself up as in Figure 5.9, with a straight line through your ear, shoulder, hip, knee, and ankle. In Figure 5.10 you can see how the imaginary vertical line of gravity relates to the front and back view of someone with good

FIGURE 5.10A   **FIGURE 5.10B**

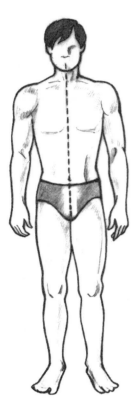 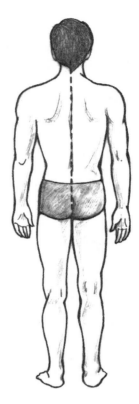

posture. In the front view (A), the shoulders are of equal height, as are the hips and knees. The head is held straight. The vertical line goes from the point of the chin to the belly button and on down through the center of the pelvis. In the view from the back (B), the spine and head are straight, not tilted or curved to the right or left.

I have worked with enough people in walking clinics to know that not all of us can have perfect posture, no matter how hard we try. Some people have misalignments and variations in their musculoskeletal systems that do not result from lack of effort on their part. Certainly some older people, especially women with osteoporosis, fall into that category.

Despite the changes that occur naturally with aging, good posture can be maintained, and for many poor posture can be improved. The American Physical Therapy Association advises: "In individuals with severe postural problems, such as poor alignments that have existed so long that structural changes have occurred, the poor posture can be kept from getting progressively worse." It recommends: "Everyone should consciously work at achieving and maintaining good posture as they grow older."

Now that you have seen what the elements of good posture are, here is a head-to-toe checklist:

1. Head straight (not tilted to either side) with chin parallel to the ground.

2. Shoulders level and loose, in line with the ears and directly over the hips.

3. Chest held moderately elevated, with the upper back erect.

4. Hips level and directly under the shoulders.

5. Knees and ankles straight and in line with hips, shoulders, and ears.

For those of you who have a posture problem, I'll bet my quail dog that getting your head up and level and keeping it that way will be your biggest challenge. It was for me, and it is for most people in my clinics. Even people with good posture tend to tilt their heads forward and look almost straight down at the ground, as in Figure 5.11A.

The most common reason given for this position is "I've got to see where I am going or I'll stumble." Sounds reasonable, but this really isn't the problem that everyone imagines. Take a look at runners; they are going much faster than walkers, yet you never see them with their heads down. Actually, it is difficult to run that way (try it). Runners' heads are up, and they are scanning the terrain ahead with their eyes. Walkers must learn to do the same.

You can see more than you think when you lower your eyes instead of your head. For instance, stand up now and put your head in the level position. Look across the room to the most distant point, as if you were scanning ahead of your walking path. Now scan with your eyes across the floor to see how close to your feet and line of travel you can see while keeping your chin parallel to the floor. Almost all people have good vision down to about 6 or 8 feet in front of them. That's really all the distance you need if you are constantly scanning ahead. Correct walking posture is shown in Figure 5.11B.

FIGURE 5.11A   **FIGURE 5.11B**

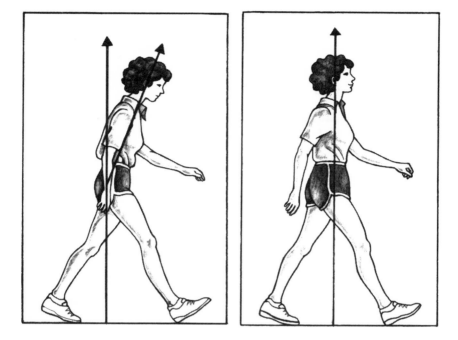

There is a fundamental reason to monitor your proper head position and to keep working on it until you can maintain it constantly. When the head tilts forward, it tends to bring the shoulders with it, and then the back is easily bent. The body tends to align itself from the top down. It is nearly impossible to have bad posture if your head is up and level. To prove this to yourself, stand up. With your head up and locked in the level position (ears in line with shoulders, chin parallel to the floor), see if you can slump your shoulders forward. As long as your head is in the proper position, your shoulders will stay there also. Good posture starts with the head.

THE STEP CYCLE AND ITS BIOMECHANICAL SUBTLETIES

Before we get into the stroll and its uses as a low-intensity exercise, a closer look at the gait we call walking will equip you to understand some of the less obvious biomechanical movements that occur on each step cycle. The more you understand your locomotion system and how it functions, the more you will appreciate what a complicated piece of biomechanical engineering you are. Everyone who owns some complex piece of high-tech equipment, or perhaps a well-engineered automobile, and who thoroughly understands and appreciates how it functions will tend to use it and conscientiously maintain it. Perhaps when you know more about your body and its locomotion system, you will do likewise.

Over the years I have looked for a well-researched book that examines the walking gait in minute detail. Dr. Lovejoy told me about such a book, appropriately entitled *Human Walking*, by Verne T. Inman, M.D., Ph.D.; Henry J. Ralston, Ph.D.; and Frank Todd. Dr. Inman was one of the pioneers in the use of electromyography (measuring the electric currents associated with muscular action) in the analysis of muscle function. The text of *Human Walking* is highly technical; it was written primarily for orthopedic doctors and other medical professionals. Nevertheless, I was able to mine a wealth of information out of it about the movements of our muscles and limbs during each step cycle; how our hips, shoulders, and legs rotate; how the foot and ankle move when we load our weight onto them; and what happens to all of these when we introduce speed into our walking gait.

In the introduction Dr. Inman states, "The mastering of the erect bipedal type of locomotion is a relatively prolonged affair and appears to be a learned process, not the result of inborn reflexes." He compares a crawling infant with a quadruped as it uses one limb to advance and the other three as support. This tripod-type stability is lost when the infant tries to rise to a bipedal position and walk. Parents and grandparents marvel as the baby takes its first few unaided, faltering steps and cringe with apprehension when it takes a few falls. As Dr. Inman points out, it is easy to observe that walking is a learning process for the baby. This does not seem to be true for the running gait, however. After slowly learning to walk, the young child quickly and instinctively runs. Survival is also an instinct, and that is why I refer to running as our survival gait.

Because walking is a learned activity, it is not surprising that each of us has certain peculiarities in our walk. You can sometimes recognize a friend by his or her manner of walking, even from a great distance. The late John Wayne had a distinctive walk that was often imitated by impressionists. Dr. Inman observes: "Tall, slender people walk differently from short, stocky people and alter their manner of walking when wearing shoes with different heel heights." He also states, "A person walks differently when exhilarated than when mentally depressed," and concludes, "Any serious description of human walking should attempt an explanation of the dissimilarities as well as the similarities."

Upper-body sway, for instance, varies with individuals. We all have this sway to some degree. It is caused by placing the lead foot wide from the track of the back foot at heel plant. As your weight is loaded onto that foot, you will list to that side. Babies learning to walk tentatively place their feet wide for stability and have a noticeable upper-body sway. We call them toddlers. If you are walking closely side by side with a friend and you are out of step, most likely your shoulders will bump because of upper-body sway. Get in step and they won't bump, because you will both be swaying in the same direction at the same time. As you learn to increase your walking pace, you will find that excessive upper-body sway is a hindrance.

According to Dr. Inman, the pelvis "becomes a suitable structure to separate the body into upper and lower parts which behave physically differently during walking." He points out that, when walking at moderate speeds, "the pelvis lists, rotates, and undulates and the arms swing out of phase with the pelvis and legs." The upper and lower body rotate in different directions as our counterbalancing mechanism for stability. As Dr. Lovejoy pointed out, being upright and walking on two legs is biomechanically complex.

If you have ever walked behind someone in a pair of tight jeans, "pelvic rotation and undulation" probably became obvious. Dr. Inman observes that at a moderate pace your pelvis rotates approximately 4 degrees to either side of your vertical line of gravity. He adds, "As your speed increases, the pelvic rotation increases markedly." The pelvis does something else when you are walking; it lists downward on the side opposite the weight-bearing leg. The hardworking abductor muscles, which you learned about in Chapter 2, kept the body from tilting over when we became upright, but the body still has a list caused by the weight of the torso bearing down on the unsupported side. People who are extremely obese not only track wide for stability but also have considerable upper-body sway and pelvic list as their locomotion systems struggle to accommodate their excess weight.

Dr. Inman and his colleagues carefully researched the biome-

chanical subtleties of the human walking gait, and you will encounter them as you learn about the various walking intensities.
As Dr. Inman points out, *"Every feature of walking changes when
walking speed changes."* Some of the movements of the limbs and
muscles that function reasonably well at a slow pace take on different characteristics as the pace quickens. Being aware of this and
understanding how to adjust for increased speed will help you
become a smoother, better walker.

Let's start slowly and work our way up:

STROLLING—LOW INTENSITY

You've stretched, you are standing erect with the proper posture,
and you are ready to take the first step to start your lifetime
exercise-walking program. I am purposely going to restate what I
said in the previous chapter: if you are going to make any mistakes
when exercising, always err on the conservative side. Start slowly
and avoid unnecessary discomfort; don't stress your cardiovascular
system before it is ready.

If you start right, one of the many beauties of walking is that
you can go from a sedentary, overweight lump all the way to a
lean, mean race walker (if that is your goal) without one day of
soreness or injury. If you are in a totally unfit, sedentary condition,
then you should definitely start at the strolling pace.

As stated in Chapter 4, the stroll is a low-intensity pace that
ranges in speed from a 30-minute mile to an 18-minute mile. Within
that range, you will automatically find a walking comfort zone. It
will be determined by your age, state of unfitness, and how much
excess weight you are carrying.

In the monthly walking clinics I conduct at the Cooper Wellness
Program, I have found that the older and heavier the walkers are,
regardless of sex, the more slowly they must start. A 30-minute
mile is quite a challenge, and some can't go a mile at any pace.
But that's okay. From that tortoiselike start, I have seen people
combine desire with determination to achieve uncommon success.
I enjoy working with these slow starters because I will never forget
when I was fat and sedentary. Don't be discouraged if you are in
this condition. Desire and determination are far more important
than speed at this stage.

Before you take your first step, let's establish how long it and
all of the other steps you take from now on should be. In other

words, what should your stride length be? The definition of *stride* in the dictionary is "to walk with long steps." In common usage, however, when people say they were "striding along," they usually mean they were walking with some determination but with normal steps. Throughout the book, I will use *stride* in this context also.

The question of step or stride length comes up in every one of my walking clinics, and there seem to be differing opinions about it. The correct stride length for you is determined by the length of your legs, the length of your hamstrings, and the law of physics that governs a pendulum.

Here is how your legs work and how they determine *your* normal stride length. If you recall the anatomy lesson in Chapter 2, the femoral head of the upper leg is attached at the pelvis in a ball-and-socket arrangement. This is the pivotal point your leg swings from, and the length of your leg from there to the ground is the main determinant of your stride length. The leg swings back and forth like a pendulum—which it is. The law of physics that governs a pendulum says that long pendulums have longer arcs than short pendulums. It follows, then, that if you have long legs you will have a longer stride than someone with short legs. When dealing with the human body, however, there always seem to be exceptions, and there are a couple to this point.

First, whatever degree of forward rotation you have in your pelvis will add to your stride length. For the stroll, brisk walk, or aerobic walk, let your pelvic rotation do what comes naturally. Do not try to exaggerate it. In Chapter 9 we will examine closely the effect of intentional forward pelvic flexion in race walking.

Stride length can also be influenced by the hamstring muscles. They will keep your leg from swinging its normal arc if they are shorter than they should be. I said it earlier, but I can't say it often enough: muscles that aren't used lose their flexibility and functionality. This is especially true for people 50 and older. Because of short hamstrings, many older people walk with abnormally short strides; some only shuffle. They can remedy this problem by regular stretching and regular walking.

There is an easy way for you to get an idea of what your stride length should be. Stand next to a wall or chair for balance, with all your weight on one leg. Tilt a bit toward your weight-bearing side so that your unweighted leg can clear the floor when it passes under your body. Hold your foot flat with your knee locked on the unweighted leg and let it swing freely, but don't *force* it forward. You will notice that your leg stops in front of you automatically, and that it stops at about the same point every time. Now stop your leg at the exact end of its forward swing and slowly plant your heel on the ground as you push off with your other foot. If you don't have short hamstrings, this is your normal stride length. If you take a few steps of this length, they should feel comfortable and effortless.

To get a taste of what happens when you try to lengthen your stride beyond what it should be, repeat the foregoing procedure, except on the forward swing do force your leg beyond the point at which it automatically stops. Now slowly plant your heel and push off with your other foot. When the swing of your foot is forced beyond its normal arc, your center of mass will drop farther than it should because your foot is too far in front of you when it makes ground contact. This causes an exaggerated, unrhythmic, up-and-down action. Take a few steps like this and you can feel it. When exercise walking, you are using your muscles and joints well within their normal range of motion. Properly done, walking always produces a smooth, fluid, natural, rhythmic movement.

Before we leave the issue of stride length, let's put the big myth about tall people being able to walk faster than short people to rest once and for all. I wish I had a quarter for every time someone in my clinics has said to me, "Well, you can walk faster than I can because you're taller." If this were the case, Wilt Chamberlain and Kareem Abdul-Jabbar should have been champion race walkers as well as champion basketball players.

To resolve this old canard, we have to go back to physics class. The law governing pendulums says that long pendulums swing *slower* than short pendulums. It is true that someone 6 feet tall will have a longer stride length than someone 5 feet tall, but if both are of equal athletic ability, the 5-footer will be able to take more strides than the 6-footer. Walking speed is determined more by stride frequency than by stride length.

A good example of this is my friend little (she hates that adjective) Wendy Sharp. I recruited her for NaturalSport's women's race-walking team. Wendy is a contender for the 1992 U.S. Olympics race-walking team. Although she claims she is 5 feet, 1½ inches tall, the top of her head is about level with my elbow.

As short as she is, Wendy can walk a mile in 7 minutes or less, and I wouldn't last 100 yards if I tried to keep up with her. I obviously have a longer stride, but she has a much greater stride frequency. Most of the world-champion men race walkers are closer to 5 feet, 9 inches than they are to 6 feet. The champion women walkers are of average height. None are amazons. I'll show you how to increase your stride frequency in the next chapter, but right now it's time to stroll.

Your Comfort Zone

The important thing for beginning exercise walkers to remember is to let the walking gait find its own strolling comfort zone, which will vary with the individual. Some people starting from sedentary can tolerate more exercise quicker than others. This can be a problem for husbands and wives, or for friends or neighbors, who want to start a walking program together. If both are sedentary but one is just a little overweight and the other is extremely overweight, the lighter walker may be comfortable at a 20-minute-mile pace while the heavier walker struggles to keep up. The danger in this situation is that the overweight walker may be putting too much stress on his or her cardiovascular system. It is also counterproductive for the faster walker to reduce the intensity of his or her walk for a slower walker.

By definition, strolling is a low-intensity physical exercise. Even so, I have worked with many people who felt as if they were climbing Pikes Peak as they struggled through their first mile in 25 or 30 minutes. If you are at this level, just hang in there and keep plugging away, because I have also had the pleasure of seeing those people cruising along at a brisk 15-minute-mile pace a few months later. Find your own comfort zone and stay with it until you improve your level of fitness. Above all, don't try to keep up with a faster walker until you are physically ready. The stroll is the entry-level walk for people with great variations of unfitness.

Strolling Objectives

Your two primary objectives with the strolling pace are, in order of importance: (1) achieve your goal for frequency; (2) achieve your goal for duration in terms of either minutes or miles. Intensity of exercise is not a consideration with the stroll, even though a walker who is struggling along at a 30-minute mile may think the 20-minute stroll is light-years away. I can assure this walker that he or she will see the day when the 20-minute mile not only isn't a challenge but may actually be boring, as our strollers in the walking study found. If this occurs, all you have to do is pick up the pace a bit. Happily, at that point your body will be ready for the increased physical challenge.

Work on your frequency and duration together—but slowly. If five days a week is your goal—and it's a good one—try to get in a little each day. It is better to go often for short walks than infrequently for long ones. Frequency adds to your discipline, and the sooner you make time every day for your walk, the sooner you will be on your way to an increased quality of life.

I vividly remember trying to make this every-day point in a walking clinic by using the comparison of the need to brush our teeth every day. I feel so strongly about the merits of exercise walking and the physical evils of being sedentary that in my lectures I sometimes pace back and forth and become almost evangelistic. On this particular day, I stopped, planted my feet, gave the class a hellfire-and-brimstone look, and with a demanding voice asked, "Would any of you even *think* of going a day without brushing your teeth?" An old guy off to my left got up, pulled out his uppers and lowers, and with a gummy smile waved them at me and the class. I went to my knees laughing, and a middle-aged, heavyset woman next to him laughed so hard that she lost control of her bladder. Believe me, I'll never forget that clinic.

The stroll is the perfect pace to help you reach your duration goal. Three miles a day, which was recommended by the President's Council on Physical Fitness, is the goal I think is the most sustainable and effective over the long term. Covering this distance at a stroll, particularly a slow stroll, takes considerable time. But, in the early stages of your walking program, you must allow for it so that you don't overload your physiological system. Once you can do 3 miles at a comfortable strolling pace, you'll be ready to work on intensity.

In addition to reaching your frequency and duration goals with the stroll, you should use this pace to establish firmly the proper walking posture. Most slow walkers tend to amble along in a slouched posture. Once your fitness improves and your initial slow pace is no longer a physical challenge, you will naturally want to increase your speed—and you should. The faster you walk, however, the more important correct posture becomes. The stroll is the ideal pace to put good walking habits in place.

I find that the tendency to tilt the head forward and slump the shoulders is the most difficult bad posture habit to break. Until you get your proper walking posture firmly in place, say to your-self, "Hips forward, shoulders back, chin up . . . hips forward, shoulders back, chin up . . . hips forward, shoulders back, chin up." Repeat it in cadence with your steps. As you walk faster, speed it up and repeat it over and over like a mantra. You will probably find that correcting a forward-tilted head is your biggest posture problem. Work on it. If I can do it, *anyone* can do it.

One final thing: don't walk with your hands in your pockets. Let them hang loose at your sides and swing back and forth freely in a relaxed manner. You don't have to swing them vigorously when strolling; that comes later. The arms counterbalance your leg and pelvic movements, however, and add to the rhythm of your walk. The stroll is the most accommodating pace to practice your posture, technique, and rhythm. When you've got all of that together and have hit your goals for frequency and duration, you are ready to move up to the brisk pace.

BRISK WALKING—MODERATE INTENSITY

The brisk walk—18- to 14-minute miles—is the pace that most long-term exercise walkers use. It delivers enough cardiovascular improvement and caloric expenditure for the time spent to be with-out question the best all-around exercise. On a risk-reward basis for all healthy people who do not have a physical impairment in their walking gait, it can't be beat.

Dr. Kenneth Cooper believes that the importance of consistency in exercise is far greater than intensity. The preoccupation with intensity of exercise since fitness awareness began about 15 years ago has turned many people off. High-impact aerobics is a dead issue, and the jogging craze is over the hill. Dr. Cooper, one of the earliest proponents of jogging and running, now firmly says, "Walk more, run less."

Intensity is still a major factor, however, in any exercise or training program. But we now know that the intensity of exercise an individual needs for a meaningful contribution to his or her cardiovascular fitness, health, and quality of life is much less than an athlete needs when training for a specific sport. The brisk pace fulfills this intensity need beautifully.

The brisk pace is rated as a moderate-intensity exercise, and because of this it has great sustainability for people of all ages—even into the eighties. Equally important, it delivers an adequate amount of *perceived exertion* for most people. By this I mean that brisk walkers feel so physically and mentally challenged that they do not become bored. Each walk is a rewarding experience for mind and body. If you recall in Chapter 4, Dr. Duncan had to put down a minor revolt with some of our 20-minute-mile strollers in the walking study because their walks became monotonous. They were no longer physically and mentally challenged by the strolling pace. Conversely, we didn't have any complaints from the 15-minute-mile brisk walkers.

To move up to the brisk pace, the walker must become aware of the importance of the role that the arm swing plays in accelerating the walking gait. It is easy to walk at the strolling pace with one's arms totally inactive, but that is why I reminded you to keep them out of your pockets. Walking with your hands in your pockets is a bad habit you will now have to break.

Arm Swing

Just like the legs, the arms are compound pendulums, and their pivotal points are the shoulders. The arms as pendulums also have a natural arc to their swing, depending on their length from the shoulder socket to the hand. Knowing how to implement a coordinated arm swing with an increased leg swing becomes important from this point on—especially if you want to move beyond the brisk walking pace.

To check your arm swing, stand up and assume the correct posture with your feet directly under your hips. With your shoulders relaxed and your arms hanging loosely at your sides, swing them back and forth, alternating the right and left arm as if you were walking. Get a full, vigorous swing, but don't try to force either arm beyond the point that feels natural, especially on the front swing.

If you swing your arms for a few seconds, you will develop a rhythm and a distance of travel on the front and back swing that feel as if each arm is in a groove. You will see that your arm on the front swing stops at about the same point every time. The same is true on the back swing. Your arm pendulum has found its arc of travel, based on the length of the arm, and to some extent the looseness and flexibility of your shoulder joint and arm muscle attachments.

When you stop your arm at the end of its arc on the front swing, notice that it has come slightly *across* your body. It should not, under any circumstance, come across the vertical line of gravity. If it does, you will be getting too much sideways motion, which distorts the arm swing's counterbalancing role relative to the legs.

I have observed some people who swing their arms straight out, parallel to their leg swing. This has an artificial, military look to it. Such an arm swing may work for the stroll and brisk paces, but, as you will find out in the next chapter, it will definitely limit your ability to accelerate beyond brisk, if that is your goal. Try to find that groove where your arm comes slightly across your body but not across your vertical line of gravity.

You probably have not paid much attention to the biomechanics of your walking gait up until now—at least most people haven't. Whether you have noticed it or not, your arms alternate with your legs on each step when you walk fast. For example, as your right leg swings forward, your left arm swings forward and vice versa. How much the arm swing actually contributes to forward propulsion will be discussed in detail in the next chapter. For now, I will let you decide for yourself that a good, vigorous arm swing helps you move along smartly.

On your next walk, pick a point about 40 yards away, put your hands in your pockets (preferably pants pockets, as opposed to jacket pockets), and see how fast you can comfortably and rhythmically walk the distance. Then take your hands out of your pockets and, with your arms swinging fully extended and vigorously as you have just practiced, see how fast you can walk back. I can predict that there will be a significant difference in the rhythm of your walk and your ability to walk faster with seemingly less effort. From now on your arm swing becomes an important ally to your leg swing as you attempt to increase your pace.

So far in this chapter we have established what your full natural stride length and your full natural arm swing should be. As a brisk walker, you now put them together, and the faster you make them swing, the faster you go. Your increased pace should be smooth, rhythmic, and comfortable. Don't force a fast pace by losing your erect posture or by excessive arm swing that isn't in sync with your leg swing. The minute you start to feel awkward, slow down, relax a bit, and smooth out your walk, then gradually pick up the pace again.

FIGURE 5.12A   **FIGURE 5.12B**

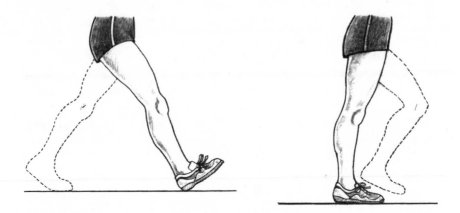

Straight-Leg Swing

A nice, rhythmic walking style with a low center of gravity and proper posture is the technique you want for the brisk pace, and, if you intend to progress to the aerobic walk, it is absolutely essential. Without it, you wouldn't have a prayer in a race walk. The brisk pace is slow enough to expand your walking technique easily and fast enough to experiment with it and perfect it.

Most good fast walkers use the straight-leg technique at heel plant. By this I mean that when your swing leg comes forward it should be fully extended and straight at the knee as the heel is placed on the ground. When your back foot pushes off and forces your body forward over that leg, keep it straight as it passes under you and becomes the trailing leg. The proper technique is shown in Figure 5.12.

In Figure 5.12A, the walker is in the double-stance phase, that brief moment when the front heel has made contact with the ground and the back toe has not yet left the ground. Notice that the lead leg is completely straight at the knee. Notice also that it is still straight at the knee as it passes under the body in Figure 5.12B.

Some people tend to walk with high bent-knee action on their lead leg. This causes them to land on the sole of their foot and to bob up and down. If they try to walk fast in this manner, they do more bobbing than going forward. If their knee is bent when it

FIGURE 5.13

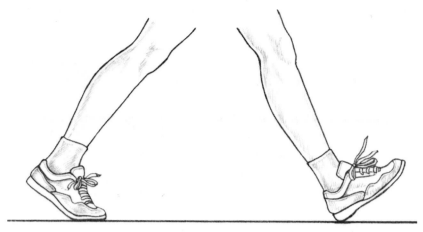

passes under them, they have that old Groucho Marx look, as if they were doing a fast creep.

The chances are that your leg is already fairly straight at heel plant and as it passes under your body. As they start to walk faster, however, some people tend to pick up speed by bending the knees. This happens most often as walkers try to move into the aerobic pace. If you see people walking fast—or attempting to—with their knees bent, they are probably doing a light flat-footed run instead of a fast walk. Their locomotion systems are using more elastic energy from their muscles instead of the lifting and falling mechanical energy of their leg pendulums. They are using a sort of hybrid gait that denies them the best benefits of either a good run or a fast walk. Check your leg swing and work on keeping your leg straight through the entire step cycle, from heel plant to weight bearing to toe-off.

Heel Plant to Toe-Off

As the heel makes contact with the ground, the forefoot and toes should be up at a comfortable angle (see Figure 5.13). Some race-walking coaches advise that the angle between the ground and the bottom of the foot be 45 degrees. Technically that may be okay, and if you progress to race walking you may want to try it. For an exercise walker, however, it is more important simply to get the toes up at a good, comfortable angle. Bringing the toes up at heel plant eliminates landing on the sole of the foot and clumping along in an awkward manner.

In addition to stride length and the straight-leg swing, the way you load your body weight onto your foot after heel plant will determine how smooth and rhythmic your walk will be. As the foot is lowered after heel plant, it should not slap down flat from heel to toe but should settle in smoothly with a slight emphasis on the outside (lateral) edge.

Biomechanically, the foot is quite complex (we will look at it in more detail in Chapter 10). For now, another one of my little experiments will clearly show you how your foot functions as you put your weight on it in a walking step. If you aren't at home as you are reading this, you may have to wait until you get there to try this experiment.

Take off your shoe and sock on one foot. For balance, it might be best to stand next to a chair. Put your sockless foot out in front of you with your heel on the floor and your toes up as if you had just taken a step and made floor contact at heel plant. Have your other foot slightly behind you, flat on the floor and bearing weight.

Now slowly elevate the heel of your back foot, as if you are starting to toe off. Let your front foot settle onto the floor gently and naturally until it is flat and you have transferred all your weight to it. Keep the toes of your back foot in contact with the floor. Reverse and transfer your weight onto your back foot again by letting the heel settle back down onto the floor as your front toes rise to their original position.

Repeat this process several times, slowly rocking back and forth while watching the action of your sockless foot as you load your weight onto it. Unless you have an abnormality in your foot—and many people do—it should naturally settle onto the floor from your heel to your toes with a slight bias to the outside edge. It should not come straight down, with your big toe making contact with the floor first. In fact, the big toe should touch the floor last. As your full weight comes down onto the foot, you can see that the forefoot noticeably widens and that your toes spread slightly.

For proper foot placement, the foot should land straight in line from heel plant to toe-off. Some people have their toes pointed in at toe-off—a condition commonly referred to as pigeon-toed. Others walk with one or both feet splaying out. Carol walks with her left foot tracking perfectly straight and her right foot splaying out about 10 degrees. She has tried to break herself of it but can't seem to get the foot to track straight permanently.

By the time people reach adulthood, they will probably walk for the rest of their lives in the way that their feet are tracking. Most have adapted to it and do quite well. In my clinics I don't try to change them because, as Dr. Inman points out, "There are great dissimilarities in the walking gait." You should know, however, that foot placement that deviates, whether in or out, much from proper alignment will affect your biomechanical efficiency as you try to increase your pace. Someone who toes in or splays out noticeably may find it difficult to walk much faster than a brisk pace. I have never seen a good race walker with that kind of foot placement.

By now you are probably wondering how you are going to remember all the nuances involved with something supposedly as simple as walking. It will be easier than you think. I suspect you are probably not very far off on many of them. In my clinics I find that most people have pretty good technique and only need to brush up on a point or two.

When something you are doing almost unconsciously is broken down biomechanically, it sometimes seems to become mentally and physically complicated. A few people put too much thought into it and try to micro-manage their walking gait. That usually leads to a stiff, unrelaxed walker. Get out, start walking, and check yourself out; you may be a natural, and all you have to do is keep going.

In order of importance, you should concentrate on (1) posture; (2) technique (leg stride and foot action); and (3) rhythm. Try to develop a fluid, smooth gait. Observe other walkers. You will see great variations of the walking gait—some people with heads bobbing up and down, others seeming to lurch from side to side. Then you will see a walker who moves with it all together in one coordinated, flowing stride.

Starting with the stroll and working up to the fast end of the brisk pace, a sedentary person can develop a good, moderate level of fitness—and this is all many people need or want. Others, however, want the benefits of an aerobic workout, and they are willing to put the necessary intensity into their exercise to achieve the higher aerobic fitness level.

The top end of the brisk pace is subaerobic for a fit individual. Consequently, most people are told to switch to another form of exercise, such as running, to get the intensity necessary to attain aerobic fitness or to accelerate caloric expenditure. As you learned in the last chapter, this is no longer necessary. Aerobic walking can take you as far up the fitness ladder as you want to go.

6 AEROBIC WALKING

Aerobic walking involves making one simple change in your arm swing that enables you to accelerate your walk from the brisk 15-minute-mile pace to a 12-minute mile or faster. The results are spectacular for weight loss, cardiovascular fitness, stress relief, and increased energy. By walking aerobically, you'll burn as many calories as a jogger and get a complete head-to-toe workout. Aerobic walking uses all the major muscle groups in the upper and lower body in a nonimpact, dynamic, rhythmic action, which is exactly what an ideal exercise should do.

Aerobic walking is a high-intensity exercise but one you can engage in without the concern for injury that goes with most other high-intensity exercises, such as running. When my first walking book was completed, I had the dilemma of choosing a title. Since it focused on walking at a pace that would put your heart into the recognized aerobic-training range, and since aerobic exercise is so widely recommended, it seemed to make sense to call it *Aerobic Walking*. This designation also helps to simplify identifying the other walking intensity levels. High-intensity aerobic walking is easily distinguished from the moderate and low intensities of brisk walking and strolling.

"Is walking an aerobic activity?" was the question posed by Dr. James Rippe and several coauthors in a January 1989 article in *Practical Cardiology* entitled "The Cardiovascular Benefits of Walking." Dr. Rippe, a cardiologist, is also clinical director of the University of Massachusetts Medical School Center for Health, Fitness, and Human Performance. He has probably done more than any other doctor to publicize and promote walking as the most beneficial exercise. The walking movement needs more Dr. Rippes.

In the article Dr. Rippe pointed out: "Many physicians believe that walking is adequate exercise for elderly or cardiac-rehabilitation patients, but lacks sufficient intensity for younger, perhaps more fit, individuals." He is absolutely correct. Not only do many physicians believe this, but so do most exercise physiologists and others involved in fitness. Dr. Rippe cited a study conducted at the Exercise Physiology Laboratory at the University of Massachusetts Medical Center that complements the study in Chapter 4 done at the Institute for Aerobics Research. In Dr. Rippe's study, highly fit young *men* between the ages of 22 and 39 were able to maintain their heart rates in the aerobic-training range while walking for 30 minutes. The men averaged 5.3 miles per hour (about 11-minute, 20-second miles), whereas the women in our study averaged 12-minute miles. Since the men started out "highly fit," it is understandable that they would have to walk faster to elevate their heart rates.

Between the two studies, however, it has now been established that gender is not a factor in walking intensity for aerobic fitness. Both men and women will incur an aerobic-training effect by walking within about a 1-minute proximity to the 12-minute-mile pace. Younger, fit walkers may have to walk a little faster; older walkers may be well within their age-related aerobic-training range by walking a little slower.

The answer to Dr. Rippe's question "Is walking an aerobic activity?" is a resounding *yes!* There are a couple of qualifiers, however. First, you must walk at a pace that is equal to slow jogging. Second, to walk this fast requires an altered arm swing. Confusion seems to arise when someone deviates from what is perceived as "normal walking," and too many in the fitness field are apt to call any such change "race walking." Since race walking is not well understood or widely viewed as a major track and field event in this country, some people shy away from altering their walking form.

In Chapter 9 I will cover all the adjustments to the walking gait required for one to become a competitive race walker. In *Aerobic Walking* I listed these adjustments and suggested that aerobic exercise walkers use them as well. I retract that suggestion now, because most people can't master the technique without considerable coaching and practice, but, more important, because it is not necessary.

I learned the race-walking technique when I was researching my first book and assumed it was required to achieve a walking pace fast enough to get an aerobic workout. That is not the case. The experience of working with thousands of people in walking clinics over the past five years has proven to me that one simple change of the arm swing is all that is necessary to accelerate your walking speed from a brisk pace to an aerobic 12-minute mile or faster. This is all that I taught the women aerobic walkers in the walking study at the Institute for Aerobics Research. They walked magnificently and hit the upper end (86 percent) of their aerobic-training range consistently.

THE BENT-ARM-SWING TECHNIQUE

Perhaps the most difficult message to get across in a walking clinic is the relative importance of a vigorous bent-arm swing to increase walking speed. It raises this question: If the walking-propulsion muscles are in the legs, then how do the arms make you go faster? When stride frequency is increased, the arm swing (in its counterbalancing role) must increase also. If the arms do not keep up with the legs, the entire walking gait becomes out of sync and labored; speed is then difficult, if not impossible, to achieve and maintain.

Dr. Inman states: "Walking is a complex integrated activity with multiple factors interacting simultaneously." This truism takes on new meaning as you try to increase your walking speed. The interaction of the arms and legs becomes more apparent. The biomechanical role the arms play in walking at a stroll is minimal. At that pace, you can even walk comfortably with your hands in your pockets. If you took the 40-yard walking test in the last chapter and tried to walk fast that way, however, you found doing so was not only uncomfortable but actually restricted your ability to stride out more quickly with a natural leg swing.

Walking at the brisk pace with the arms fully extended and swinging freely at your sides, it is easy to get a smooth, comfortable leg swing and to maintain your speed. The brisk pace tops out at about a 14-minute mile, however, or at least becomes so labored that it is uncomfortable to maintain because your fully extended arms cannot swing fast enough to serve as counterbalancers.

When you are walking at a pace that is equivalent to a slow jog, your arms must be able to swing fast enough to complement and counterbalance the increased leg swing. The long, extended-arm pendulum must be shortened so that you can swing it faster. The compound feature of your arm pendulum permits you to bend it at the elbow and bring the forearm up so that it forms a 90-degree angle with your upper arm. In effect, you have shortened your arm so that you can swing it faster. By locking the angle at the elbow so that your forearm does not flop up and down, you allow it to swing in a neutral arc. Discounting the slight effect of the weight of the forearm, you are essentially swinging pendulums as long as the distance from the bottom of your elbow to your shoulder socket. The shortened arm pendulums will now swing as fast as you can make your legs go.

A way to feel the difference in swing frequency is to stand with one arm fully extended and locked rigid at the elbow. Swing your long-arm pendulum back and forth as fast as you can within its normal swing range. Don't swing it on the forward swing any farther than you would when walking briskly.

Now bring your forearm up to a 90-degree angle at the elbow and pump your upper arm back and forth as fast as you can. Notice how much faster it swings. A metronome, used by musicians to maintain a slow or fast beat, works the same way. With the weight farthest from the point of swing it goes slowest, but, as the weight is moved closer to the point of swing, the beat goes faster.

Your forearm, wrist, and hand hanging down fully extended put most of the weight of your arm *below* the elbow. This makes your arm act like the slow metronome. The simple act of elevating this weight, even with the elbow, permits your arms to swing faster.

If you have progressed through the frequency, duration, and intensity sectors of your walking program and can walk 3 miles in 45 minutes without undue physical stress, you are a prime candidate for aerobic walking. You have achieved a moderate level of fitness and are already contributing to your longevity and quality of life.

Dr. Rippe's article pointed out that there is no epidemiologic evidence that decreased coronary heart disease is related to walking intensity. Walking faster, however, will increase your cardiovascular fitness, which, according to Dr. Rippe, includes "a decrease in resting heart rate, increase in maximal oxygen consumption (VO_2 max) and the ability to accomplish a given task at a lower percentage of VO_2 max." Aerobic walking will make your heart more fit to function, but, as was pointed out in Chapter 1, there is a distinct difference between fitness and health.

I am not trying to dissuade you from walking aerobically. I do it every day, as does my wife, and we find it the perfect aerobic exercise. It is a quick way to burn extra calories, and the increased cardiovascular fitness from it gives us a higher energy level. The intensity component of exercise walking, however, should be added only if you can consistently maintain frequency and duration. If you are game, then let's give it a whirl.

Some interesting things happen to some people when they start to walk fast with their arms bent at the elbow. Everyone has heard the old saw about people who are "so uncoordinated they can't walk and chew gum at the same time." Don't laugh; you might feel like this yourself for a bit. You have walked your whole life, your arms flopping along at your sides, without thinking about them. Now, with them bent, some people start to think about their arms—and sometimes strange things happen.

When the mind begins to manage the arms, which it has paid no attention to up until now, there is a tendency to swing an arm forward on the same side as the leg that is swinging forward. This creates a stilted, uncoordinated look. The walker immediately senses something is wrong but can't quite figure out what.

Men are probably tired of hearing me rave about women walkers, but, in most of the classes I have taught, more men than women have trouble with the bent-arm swing. At the Cooper Wellness Program, where the average age of the participants is 48, I find that a number of middle-aged men tend to walk like the Energizer bunny, while their wives are cruising around the track like sports cars. However, this is only a temporary problem for a few; in a matter of minutes everyone usually adapts to this minor alteration of the arm swing.

With humans, there are always exceptions, even to something

as simple as walking with your arms bent. In August 1989, I had a 42-year-old investment banker from Illinois named Larry in a walking clinic. When he used the bent-arm position and walked, his knees came up as if he were a drum major marching. When I had him drop his forearms to their natural position, his knees went down to their natural position. Larry walked as if he had strings connecting his wrists to his kneecaps. When a wrist went up, so did the knee. When we parted later that day, he was still fighting his problem. He is the only person I know of who couldn't master the bent-arm swing in a very short time.

Before you attempt to change to the bent-arm swing on your daily walk, try a little coordinating experiment at home. Stand with your head up, chin parallel to the floor, and posture erect as if you were walking, except keep your feet stationary directly under your pelvis. Let your shoulders relax and let your arms swing fully extended and vigorously, as if you were on a brisk walk. Swing them through their full normal range from front to back.

On the front swing you will notice that just as the upper arm stops its motion the forearm will continue upward and slightly across your body by bending at the elbow from the momentum of the swing. Swing the arms several times so that you are relaxed at the shoulders.

Now, while swinging the arms, slowly raise the forearms until they are at right angles to your upper arms. Keep the shoulders relaxed. Some people tend to elevate their shoulders when they elevate their forearms. Keep swinging the arms, then lower them to the extended position again. Repeat this cycle several times to see if you are equally relaxed at the shoulders whether your forearms are up or down. Sometimes, as the swing frequency is increased, coordination suffers and tightness in the shoulders develops. When you feel as relaxed and coordinated with the forearms up as down, increase the frequency of their swing to see how fast you can move them back and forth.

I find it is easier for most people to get the hang of the bent-arm swing by swinging their arms while standing—preferably in front of a mirror—than when out walking. If you swing them properly, the upper arms will not travel any farther than they did when the arms were fully extended. However, because the forearm now projects in front of you, it seems as if it does go farther.

To prove that it doesn't, in my clinics I put a Day-Glo-orange armband around my elbow to focus attention on the length of the

FIGURE 6.1   FIGURE 6.2

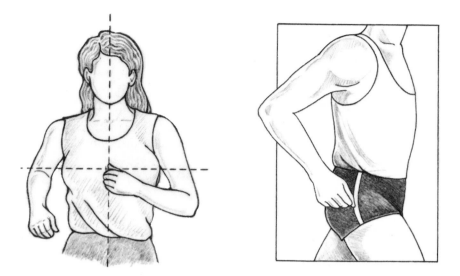

arc it travels while the arm is swinging fully extended. As I raise my forearm to the 90-degree angle, the arc of the swing remains exactly the same.

If the forearm is not brought all the way up to a 90-degree angle, you are swinging a partially shortened pendulum that will put some drag on your ability to achieve the maximum frequency of your arm swing. Many people tend to let their forearms hang below their elbows. It is always better to bend the forearm a little bit above the elbow than to let it hang below.

With the forearm in its new position, a couple of tendencies occur in most people's arm swings. One is to swing the arms too high on the front swing and not far enough on the back swing. Figure 6.1 shows the arm in its proper position at the end of the front swing.

Let your hand form a loose fist. If you clench it, you will tighten the muscles in the arm. The arms should hang loosely from the shoulders so that the forearms pass close to your body. If you are wearing a sweatshirt or jacket, it is okay for the sleeve to brush your body lightly. At the end of the front swing, your hand should be slightly across the front of your body, but not across the center line of gravity as shown in Figure 6.1, and the hand should never go higher than the line across the top of your breast.

On the back swing, your loose fist should come to about your midbuttocks, as in Figure 6.2. Most people tend to stop short on the back swing. Try bringing your loose fist back to just behind the seam of your pants and you will probably feel a slight pull at your shoulder. Hold your loose fist still at your hip at the end of its back-swing arc for a couple of seconds, then quickly relax the shoulder muscles. The shortened arm pendulum will naturally drop forward, and it only takes a little muscle power to increase the speed of its forward swing. Concentrate on putting muscle power into your back swing. If your arm pendulum gets a full, vigorous back swing, the front swing will almost take care of itself.

My experience in walking clinics is that about 25 percent of people pick up the bent-arm swing immediately, another 25 percent pick it up in a matter of minutes, and the remaining 50 percent have to play with it for a little while. Except for Larry the banker, I have never found anyone who couldn't master it in a couple of walks. I sure hope Larry is a better banker than he is a walker.

I will guarantee you that if you couple correct posture with your normal stride length and the bent-arm-swing technique, you can walk at the top end of your aerobic-training range. You do not have to change the normal way your legs and hips move. This is not race walking; it is aerobic walking. Coordinate your faster bent-arm swing with your faster leg swing and take off.

MOVE FROM BRISK TO AEROBIC WALKING—SLOWLY

I don't want to leave you with the impression that if you simply bend your arms and swing them a little faster you will automatically go from a brisk 15-minute mile to an aerobic 12-minute mile. More important, you should not even try to do so. Pick up the pace a little at a time. If you are now walking 3 miles in 45 minutes, see if the new arm-swing technique will help you to do it in 44 minutes. That's increasing your speed by only 20 seconds a mile. Most people can do so without any discomfort or unwanted stress. Try to reduce your total walking time in small increments, such as 3 miles in 44 minutes, down to 43, down to 42, and so on, but do it over a period of weeks or months, not days.

Check your heart rate each day to see if it is in the aerobic-training range. If your heart rate is below your 65 percent training range, you aren't walking fast enough to be aerobic. If the legs and arms move faster, your heart rate will automatically increase. Equally important: if your heart rate is over your 85 percent training range, slow down. You have no need to walk faster. Your heart rate is telling you that your fitness level isn't as good as you think it is. For instance, if walking a 14-minute mile puts your heart rate over 85 percent, then increasing your speed would be a mistake. You should actually slow down a little. As your fitness level rises, your heart rate will decline; *then* you can pick up the pace of your walk. Remember: *heart rate is always more important than minutes per mile as a gauge of your fitness level.*

DOMINANT- AND SUBDOMINANT-ARM SWING

The amount the bent-arm swing adds to an exercise walker's ability to increase walking speed to a 12-, 11-, or even 10-minute mile cannot be overstated. Without it, your pace will plateau. To get the maximum benefit, the arms must swing in the groove shown in Figures 6.1 and 6.2. For the arms to be fully effective as counterbalances for the legs, they should also swing *evenly*.

It is an unusual person who can move to the bent-arm swing with the swing in both the right and left arms evenly matched. By this I mean that a person who is right-handed will have a more coordinated, vigorous swing with his or her right arm (the dominant arm) than with the left (the subdominant). Of course, the reverse is also true. I am a lefty, so my right arm is the one that requires my concentration. I have fun in my clinics telling participants whether they are right- or left-handed simply by watching their bent-arm swing. The dominant and subdominant difference is more difficult to call when the arm is fully extended. I ask people to bend their arms and pump them back and forth as if they were walking. The most obvious tip-off to the subdominant arm is that the person does not take it as far back on the back swing as the dominant arm or as far forward on the front swing. It swings midrange in a namby-pamby manner. People are often amazed at the difference between their arm swings.

You can check the difference on yourself. Place your subdominant hand firmly on the point of your dominant shoulder just above where the upper arm joins the shoulder. For example, right-handers would place their left hands on their right shoulders, and southpaws would do the opposite. Now pump the dominant arm vigorously back and forth as if you were doing the bent-arm swing. Take it clear back to the midbuttocks and as far forward as shown in Figure 6.1. After pumping it a few times to feel the coordinated vigor of the swing, reverse the procedure. With your dominant hand on your subdominant shoulder, pump this arm the same way. I have had people laugh out loud when their subdominant arm swung out where they didn't want it to go. They couldn't believe that there could be so much variance in the coordination of their arms. You may not have a lot of variance, but I suspect there will be enough to notice some difference in vigor and coordination between your arms.

This dominant, subdominant difference in arm swing is a subtlety you should be aware of so that you can continually monitor your subdominant arm to make sure you are getting a balanced arm swing. As you pick up your walking speed, it becomes more critical that each part of your musculoskeletal system be coordinated and balanced in every phase of each step cycle. If you decide to progress to race walking, a balanced arm swing is a must. It takes a while to get consistent balance in the arm swing, and even then there will be lapses.

Those of you with home video recorders, have someone take a videotape of your various walking intensities from time to time. This is an excellent way to check the progress of your walking form for posture, arm swing, foot placement, and leg action.

THE ARM-SWING DRILL

To establish the importance of the relationship of arm swing and leg speed, I run a little drill in my clinics that requires the participants to set the pace of their walk with their *arms* instead of their legs. Going a distance no longer than a basketball court, I get next to the walkers and keep shouting, "Pump your arms, pump your arms" to get them to move them as fast as they can while trying to keep their legs moving in sync.

When a walker gets his arms and legs moving in synchrony and sets the cadence of the walk by pumping the arms fast, the legs want to follow. In fact, the arms can pump so fast that the legs will want to break into a jog. There seems to be a neuromotor connection between your arms and legs that makes them want to work in unison at high speed. You may want to try this drill on

FIGURE 6.3A   **FIGURE 6.3B**

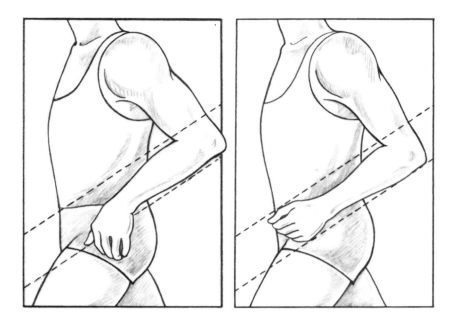

your own, but unless you can mentally force your arms to set a fast cadence and still keep your legs coordinated, you probably won't experience the effect I describe.

As part of the arm-swing drill, I also have people walk as fast as they can for about half the distance of a basketball court using the bent-arm swing. At half court in full stride, I shout, "Drop them," and have them drop their forearms quickly to the fully extended position and swing them as fast as they can while they continue walking quickly. I generally hear a few loud groans and see a few smiles as the walkers feel the drag of the fully extended arm pendulum. As one woman said, "My God, it's like dropping an anchor!" Try it yourself; you'll feel it too.

In addition to helping you walk faster, the bent-arm swing has another little plus. Many who walk several miles at a brisk pace with their arms fully extended and swinging vigorously complain of fingers swelling—sometimes so much so that the area around a ring can become painful. This pooling of blood and fluids in the fingers and hands caused by the centrifugal force of the extended arm does not occur with the bent-arm swing.

Once the forearm is brought up into the 90-degree position, it is important to keep the wrist and hand in line with the arm. Some people—women more than men—tend to let their hands flop up and down, as in Figure 6.3A. The correct position is shown in Figure 6.3B. A flopping movement at the end of the forearm transfers up the arm and affects the arm swing.

When you master the bent-arm swing and get your dominant and subdominant arms swinging with equal vigor, the only limits on how fast you can walk will be determined by your ability to maintain concentration. As your walking speed progresses beyond the 14-minute mile, you will find that if your mind wanders your speed will drop. This is a common experience as people increase their walking speed into the range of a slow jog. Over time, the amount of concentration needed diminishes, but it remains more than is required for jogging.

Walking at the aerobic pace becomes a physical *and* mental exercise because it requires a rhythmic coordination of your upper and lower body, plus the mental concentration to force your pace beyond a normal brisk walk. In Chapter 3 I called jogging a *no-brainer* exercise, and I can prove it to you. Walk as fast as you can for about 40 yards, then kick into a run *at the same pace* and see how it requires less concentration and physical effort. Running requires no mental concentration at all. Now drop back to a walk at the same pace as the run and you will immediately realize that an aerobic walk is far more challenging, both physically and mentally, than running. You also experienced the difference between gait efficiency (running) and gait *in*efficiency (walking) when you made this shift.

As testimony to the perceived difference in exertion between aerobic walking and jogging, I had to smile when I received a letter from Dr. Kenneth Cooper on a matter not related to walking. In a postscript he wrote, "I have been experimenting with race walking [he really meant aerobic walking] myself! I am now able to walk 5 kilometers [3.1 miles] averaging faster than 12 minutes per mile. For a 'confirmed runner' that is a fast walk!" You bet it is, and all runners, "confirmed" or otherwise, struggle when they try to walk fast. Dr. Cooper was referring to aerobic walking as race walking, but this is a common mistake, and I will clear up the confusion between the two in Chapter 9.

Some walkers—women more than men—find that their upper arms tire when they convert to the bent-arm swing. The combination of swinging the arms faster and holding the forearms up temporarily causes bicep fatigue. If this occurs for you, just lower your forearms enough to relieve the fatigue. After you have rested them awhile, pull them up to the 90-degree angle again until they tire. Keep repeating this fatigue-and-rest cycle during your walk, and in a few days the fatigue will be gone.

One final comment about bent arms. The first thing runners do is pull their arms up to a 90-degree angle. Do you ever see distance runners or exercise joggers with their arms hanging at their sides fully or even partially extended? Because runners are bouncing along with elastic energy, their arms play a lesser role than walkers' arms do. Even so, runners couldn't run very fast if their arms were hanging down at their sides. Try it sometime. Walkers can't walk very fast either with their arms fully extended at their sides. Aerobic walkers (and race walkers) must use their arms in a stride-for-stride vigorous pumping action in much the way sprinters do.

THE 13-MINUTE-MILE WALL

Since my book *Aerobic Walking* was published, I have gotten a good number of letters and phone calls from people who say they are using the bent-arm-swing technique but they just can't get beyond a 13-minute mile. In walking clinics that I have conducted from Boston to San Diego, the 13-minute-mile wall seems to stop a lot of aerobic walkers temporarily. To get through it becomes a matter of *mind over muscle*.

Once you get your arms and legs working in synchrony, the next challenge is to get your brain to signal your leg muscles to move as fast as you want them to. In the normal range of walking that is not a problem, but walking faster than 13-minute miles is beyond the normal range. The walking muscles must be programmed to "fire" at that intensity. The brain sends a signal out to the muscles, which are to perform a certain function, and electrical impulses within the muscles "fire." The muscles then perform their specific function. For instance, make a fist and then open and close your fist as fast as you can, a few times. That happened because your brain was sending a signal out to fire the muscles in your hand to make them contract and relax as you wanted.

I find the many similarities between our biomechanical locomotion system and the automobile fascinating. I told you about the similarities of gaits to gears in Chapter 3. There is also a similarity between the muscles "firing" by electrical impulse to move the body about and the spark plugs in a car's motor firing an electrical spark to make the fuel explode and power the pistons, which make the drive shaft and ultimately the car move.

The brain signals the muscles to get them to move by way of motor neurons. (The dictionary defines *motor neuron* as "a nerve cell that conducts impulses to a muscle"). In their book on human walking, Dr. Inman and associates state, "The response of muscles in the body depends on several factors: (1) The number of motor neurons activating the muscle at any given moment, and (2) The rates at which the various motor neurons are firing." If you want to walk faster, you have to get the signals to your muscles to fire faster. Sounds simple, but it takes some real physical effort and mental concentration.

To get beyond the 13-minute-mile wall, I teach a variation of *interval training* that runners use to increase their speed. Interval training involves fast work in short segments followed by recovery periods. For instance, a runner who competes in a mile race might run a quarter-mile interval at a faster pace than he could run the whole mile. He then slows down to a slow jog or walk for about a quarter mile to let his body recover before running a fast quarter again. A well-trained runner might repeat that cycle four to eight times in one workout session.

If you want to try a modified interval-training process, find a measured distance, like a high school quarter-mile track. Warm up for a mile, then blast off and try to walk a quarter mile in 3 minutes or less; that is the equivalent of a 12-minute-mile pace. Walk a slow, comfortable recovery quarter, then do another fast quarter. Repeat until you have done four fast quarters. Add up the times for the fast quarters, and you'll probably have a *total* time that is faster than a 13-minute mile.

By walking short, fast spurts, you actually program your brain to increase the firing of your walking muscles at speeds they are unaccustomed to. It then becomes a matter of lengthening the process. I suggest that you do only four fast and four slow sessions (alternate them) per workout and only one interval workout per week.

In the early stages of aerobic walking, concentration is almost as important as the physical ability to sustain a fast walking speed, beyond the 13-minute mile. You will find that your speed drops if your mind starts to wander. Later on, as you become an accom-

plished aerobic walker and your muscles know how t
you will not have to focus your mind on them nearl'

There is a beneficial side effect from training your '
cles to fire at a high intensity. It makes all your daily
less enervating and your normal walking pace will increase without
any more effort. On a trip to EPCOT Center at Disney World
several years ago, Carol and I were comfortably walking along
rubbernecking at all the sights when the couple we were with
hollered for us to slow down. They were about 50 yards behind
us. When I checked our speed, we were at the brisk pace, but it
was as easy and comfortable as a stroll for us. All the aerobic
walkers I know say the same thing—and so will you.

COULD IT BE SHINSPLINTS?

The one thing I can predict with certainty that will happen as you
accelerate your walk is *shin fatigue*. It generally hits most people
somewhere between a 14- and a 13-minute-mile pace, but those
who are quite a bit overweight may encounter it at slower speeds.
Shin fatigue held me back when I first tried for the 12-minute mile,
so don't be surprised or alarmed when it shows up on your walk.

Most walkers think they have shinsplints, but they don't. Happily, shinsplints are reserved for runners. In *Conquering Athletic
Injuries*, Dr. David Bernstein explains, "Shin splints are caused by
very small tears in the leg muscles at their points of attachment to
the shin." He says they result from "muscular imbalances, insufficient shock absorption, toe running, or excessive pronation of
the foot." These are running problems compounded by the foot's
impact on the ground. I have yet to find an exercise walker with
a true case of shinsplints.

It *is* common for exercise walkers who are trying to move into
the 12-minute-mile range to experience extreme fatiguing of the
big muscle that runs down the front of the lower leg, along the
shinbone. Its medical name is *tibialis anterior*, but we'll just call
it the shin muscle. Although there are other muscles in the front
of the lower leg, this is the one that is going to cause you some
temporary discomfort.

In Figure 6.4 you can see the muscle I am talking about. It is
often called the toe lifter because it is attached to the top of your
foot and pulls your forefoot toward your shin so your foot will
clear the ground as your leg swings under you. It also keeps your

FIGURE 6.4

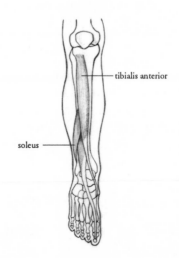

foot from flopping on the ground when you plant your heel and load your weight onto your foot.

Get to know and understand this muscle because, until you toughen it up, there will be times you will think it is on fire if you are walking faster than a 14-minute mile. You are already using this muscle in every step you take, but you are using it at a very low intensity. When you start walking at greater speeds, you use it at a higher repetition of work, and, like any of your other muscles, if it isn't conditioned for the work load, it will quickly fatigue, causing a burning sensation.

While you are seated, you can get an idea of the amount of work this muscle does. Pull your pant leg up to your knee (if you are a man or a woman in slacks) and with your heel on the floor, but slightly in front of you, pull your forefoot slowly toward your shinbone as far as you can. If you do not have fat legs, you will be able to see the muscle bulge about 4 inches below your knee. Press your fingers on the muscle at the bulge and rock your foot up and down rapidly while keeping your heel on the floor. Do this quite a few times, and you will start to feel some fatigue even while sitting.

With your foot still slightly in front of you and your forefoot *off the floor* as if you had just planted your heel taking a step, rise out of your chair and load your weight onto that heel. Feel how hard the muscle is now. The shin muscle pulls your forefoot up on every step, and at heel plant it has to work to keep your forefoot from flopping to the floor as you load your entire body weight onto the foot. The muscle is actually stretched while it is actively developing contractile tension. According to Dr. Inman, it is "engaging in a lengthening contraction." In effect, it is working two ways at the same time.

In *Aerobic Walking*, I recommended some shin-muscle exercises for conditioning, but, after several years of working with people in clinics, I have come to the belief that the best way to resolve shin muscle fatigue is to *walk it tough*. By that I mean walk at a speed that causes discomfort in the muscle, hold it as long as you can, then slow down to a pace where the discomfort disappears. Walk at that pace for about half the distance you just walked when the shin was uncomfortable, then pick up the pace and fatigue the muscle again.

In exercise physiology, this is called progression and overload. You ask the muscle to work a little harder and a little longer each time, with periods of relaxation between. Over time the shin muscle will toughen up and be able to handle the increased speed. When you get so you can go a full mile without shin fatigue, you have it whipped. You'll be able to go 3, 4, or 5 miles also. It took me about two and a half weeks to get mine in shape, but I was 56 years old. I know younger walkers who get their shin muscles toughened in a week or less. The heavier you are, the harder those shin muscles have to work, but so do the rest of your muscles. It takes an overweight person somewhat longer to get the shin muscles fit.

A FEW DOS AND DON'TS

Do keep your elbows as close to your body with the bent-arm swing as they are when your arm is fully extended and hanging at your side. Many people have a tendency to stick their elbows out when they bend their arms. But having the elbows out from the body changes the position of the upper arm at the shoulder. When you swing your arms from that position, they will go across your body and lose their effectiveness as counterbalances for your legs. I call that chicken winging.

To compare the proper elbow position with the chicken-winging position, sit erect on the edge of a chair and bend your dominant arm 90 degrees at the elbow. With your upper arm hanging loose at your side, slowly bring it back so your loosely formed fist is at your hip, then slowly bring it forward till it is out in front of you (see Figures 6.1 and 6.2). Let your arm rock slowly back and forth like that a few times. If you are totally relaxed, your elbow should be close to your body and your forearm should lightly brush your rib cage just above your waistband. Your arm should swing back and forth as if it were in a groove. That's the groove you want when you are in full stride and your arms are swinging vigorously.

Now elevate your elbow away from your body about the width of a cantaloupe so you can see the floor between your elbow and your rib cage. Slowly bring your hand back toward your hip, then forward. You will see that the hand comes across your center line of gravity and above the breast. It is automatically guided that way because, by elevating your elbow out from your body, you have changed the way the upper arm rotates from the shoulder socket. Move your arm back and forth slowly to observe the path it takes, then pump it faster a few times. You can see that if you were walking fast and chicken winging you would be getting counter-productive lateral arm movement. Keep those elbows close to the body; don't be a chicken winger.

Do keep your shoulders in a natural, relaxed position. There is a great tendency among early students of the bent-arm swing to tense the upper body around the shoulders. I see it in all of my clinics, and I myself had the problem for a few days. Relax, relax, relax.

Don't hunch your shoulders as you increase your walking speed. I also struggled with this for a couple of weeks when I was learning. There is a tendency to elevate the shoulders as you accelerate your speed. It seems as if the shoulders want to touch the earlobes. I call this the Frankenstein look, and men seem more prone to it than women. When you break into a jog, your shoulders seem to elevate just at that moment. A walker walking at the pace of a jog sometimes gets his shoulders in that position too. It may not be a problem with you, but if it is, the solution is to relax, relax, relax.

Don't walk wide. As you learned in the last chapter, placing the feet in a wide track causes upper-body sway. At slower walking speeds this is not critical; it can be accommodated up to the mid-range of the brisk pace fairly well. As you move up through the 13-minute-mile pace, though, unnecessary upper-body sway becomes counterproductive to forward progression and will affect your ability to become a smooth, fast walker. A narrow track, of 4 inches *or less* (measured as the width between the heels at their medial or inside edges at heel plant), keeps upper-body sway to a minimum.

An interesting way to observe upper-body sway is to walk with the sun behind you so that it casts your shadow directly in front of you. Walk at a brisk pace with your feet purposely tracking very wide and watch the side-to-side sway of your shoulders and head (some people walk this way all the time). Continue walking as you slowly decrease the width of your track until your feet land in a very narrow track. Upper-body sway should hardly be noticeable now.

Don't toe off until your trailing leg is well behind your pelvis. When you see people walking with their heads bobbing up and down (I call them bouncers), they are probably pushing off with their trailing feet still too close to and possibly even partially under their bodies. Remember how, when you stood with your feet under you and rotated your ankles by pushing against the floor with your forefoot, your body rose straight up. The lifting and falling action of the walking gait is exaggerated on the lifting part of the step cycle by toeing off too soon.

Although premature toe-off is not in any way injurious, it is biomechanically inefficient. It delays forward progression. It will also affect your ability to accelerate smoothly. In the stroll or brisk walk it is not a factor, but beyond a 14-minute mile it is. A narrow-track walker with the proper toe-off will be smooth and fast. A wide-track bouncer trying to walk fast will oscillate like an out-of-balance wheel on an automobile. I hate to keep harping on the gender differences between good walkers and bad, but I see twice as many wide-track men bouncers as wide-track women bouncers.

IT ISN'T RACE WALKING!

I originally felt that the complete race-walking technique was necessary to reach the aerobic range of walking. As I said earlier in this chapter, my clinical experience and that of the walking study at the Institute for Aerobics Research have since convinced me that the bent-arm swing coupled with your normal stride is all you need. Aerobic walking has only the bent-arm swing in common with race walking. Put that together with correct posture and your normal stride, and you are on your way.

When walkers develop a good, coordinated aerobic-walking technique, they really look smooth. Some women become so smooth and rhythmic in their walks that they actually look *sensual*. Look around the streets, parks, and shopping malls, and you will see more and more aerobic walkers using the bent-arm-swing technique every day.

AEROBIC WALKING CHECKLIST

This chapter has covered all the biomechanical aspects of aerobic walking and how your walking gait must be managed to move at the high-intensity level. I have thrown a lot of information at you, so here is a checklist to help you remember all the key points.

1. *Posture.* Posture is very important in the stroll and brisk paces but absolutely critical at the aerobic pace. Fatigue will set in quickly, especially in the shoulders and lower back, without proper posture. Chin up, head level, shoulders relaxed, hips in line under the shoulders, back straight, body erect. Do not compromise any of the foregoing in the interest of speed. Keep checking to make sure that your head is level and your chin is up and parallel to the ground. It is almost impossible for the shoulders to sag if your head is in the proper position. Scan the terrain ahead by lowering your eyes—not your head.

2. *Arms Bent 90 Degrees at the Elbow.* Hold your forearms up at a constant 90-degree angle at the elbows, and swing the arms from the shoulders with power and vigor in sync with your leg stride.

3. *Arm Swing.* Your forward arm swing should end with the hand slightly in front of your body (never across the center line of gravity) and no higher than the top of your breast. The back swing should go back till your loose fist is at your midbuttocks or behind the side seam of your shorts. Elbow and forearm should be close to your rib cage when they pass. Avoid chicken winging. *Complete vigorous movement of the arms through the full swing cycle is extremely important.* Make sure your subdominant arm is swinging with the same coordination and vigor as your dominant arm.

4. *Hands.* Form a loose fist. Do not clench your fist and put tension in the arm muscles. Keep your hands and wrists in straight lines with your forearms.

5. *Narrow Track.* Try to walk a narrow track, about 4 inches or less measured from the inside edge of each heel at the point of heel plant. Avoid upper-body sway caused by wide-track walking.

6. *Foot Placement.* As the heel of the lead foot is placed on the ground, the toes should be up at a comfortable angle. The forefoot should be lowered to the ground in a smooth, even manner with a *slight* emphasis on the outside edge of the foot. Avoid slapping the foot straight down from heel to toes.

7. *Straight Leg.* At heel plant, have your lead leg straight at the knee and keep it that way all the way through its weight-bearing phase as it passes under your body. Walking with high knee action is not smooth and often leads to placing the foot flat on the ground instead of with the toes up.

8. *Toe-off.* The power of the step comes from the toe-off action of the foot. Make sure your trailing leg is well behind you so that your toe-off does not cause unnecessary rise of your body, creating a bouncy look.

9. *Shoulders.* Your shoulders should be squared to your line of travel and hang relaxed. The shoulder of the arm swinging forward will tend to rotate slightly forward with it. Do not try to increase this rotation. Let your shoulders function in a natural, relaxed manner.

10. *Hip Movement.* The hip has a slight natural rotation forward with the leg swinging forward. This movement varies greatly among individuals but seems more accentuated in women than in men. Walk with your hips under your shoulders and squared to your line of travel. Let them rotate in a natural, comfortable manner. You will notice more rotation as you increase speed.

11. *Frankenstein.* Avoid hunching your shoulders as you try to walk faster. Doing so tenses your upper body and causes fatigue. It also distorts your posture and ruins your rhythm. Keep the shoulders down in their natural position and relaxed at all times.

12. *Groucho Marx.* Avoid the Groucho Marx creep by keeping your lead leg straight from heel plant to toe-off. A fast walk with bent knees ultimately converts to a flat-footed run, in which you are using elastic energy. You might as well go into a full jog.

13. *Putting It All Together.* In order of importance, concentrate on posture, technique, rhythm, and speed. When all these become one synchronized, fluid move, when you have perfect posture and are totally relaxed, when the ground flows by under your feet as you are smoothly cruising along—*then* you've got it all together.

Whether you exercise by the minute or the mile, there is no other aerobic exercise that is always accessible, injury-free, and as effective as aerobic walking.

7

THE SPECIFICITY
PRINCIPLE
AND WALKING
COMPARED WITH
OTHER EXERCISES

By now, some readers may have the opinion that I am somewhat overzealous about exercise walking. My answer to that is, You bet, I admit it! I am also confident that those who are still doubters about walking being the best exercise will share my zeal by the time this chapter is over. If not, at the very least, I will save you from some miserable exercise time and maybe save you some money—if it's not too late.

The case for exercise was made in Chapter 1, but telling people what is good for them produces only a limited response. If we did what was good for ourselves and others, there would be no smokers, no drug addicts, no alcoholics, not even a police force. We would take proper care of our bodies—we only get one—we would live by the Golden Rule, and the world would be one big healthy, peaceful place. Nice thought, but the real world doesn't work that way and never will. Bibles don't stop bloodshed, and advice about good health and exercise rarely stops those who are bent on abusing themselves.

The best I can hope to do with this book is to give you the reasons you need to exercise and hope they soak in—if not now, maybe later. If they do, then you need to know *which exercise gives you the best results for your time invested* and which exercise you are more likely to stick with. There is a babble of voices out there telling you this exercise works best, that exercise works best, and this exercise machine does more than that one. How do you sort it all out? Let's do it together and see if you come up with the same conclusions I did.

I was always looking for the easy way out before I found exercise walking. I would read an ad about some magical piece of exercise equipment that said, "fun," "burns more calories than ———," "great for the heart," "only 12 minutes a day," "effortless," and on and on. Thirty seconds after I'd straddled the dumb thing, I knew the "fun" part was a lie, and the rest didn't matter. When you get the "effortless" pitch for exercise equipment, don't waste your time. How can something that is *supposed* to take effort be effortless?

If you aren't exercising now, it is probably for one of three reasons. "I don't have the time" is the reason cited most often. "I tried exercise and became injured" is the second most frequent, and "I tried exercise and it doesn't work" is the third. I guarantee you, exercise walking will take care of numbers 2 and 3, and even number 1. People who are walkers *find* the time. Most likely you didn't find the time to do a particular exercise because you didn't like it. That's human nature. I will confess to that one a hundred times or more. Isn't it just common sense that none of us is going to premeditatedly do something we don't like for very long if we can avoid it?

It is a bit ironic that I live in Missouri, the "Show Me" state. You have every right to say "Show me." I will be glad to; in fact, it was the "show-me" approach I used on myself to compare walking with all the other exercises. I made up my mind that if I was going to take my valuable time to work up a sweat every day it had better be worthwhile.

The first thing to do for the show-me approach to exercise is establish the criteria for the *ideal lifetime exercise*. I will give you six things that I insist my exercise have, and you decide if they are equally important to you. I will list them in the order of my priorities, but you may not value them in that order. The only thing that is relevant is whether you agree that all six characteristics are essential for an exercise you expect to do for a lifetime.

LIFETIME EXERCISE CRITERIA

1. *Exercise must be natural, not boring, and somewhat enjoyable.* Everything about exercise starts and stops right here. You, me, we, they, or whoever won't stay with exercise if we dread it or if it is unnatural and mind numbing. Exercise is a tough sell; telling you it's good for you just isn't enough. It has to make you feel good physically and mentally.

2. *It must be injury free.* It was injury that mercifully ended my exercise running and forced me to find walking. Unfortunately, the majority of people who get injured doing exercise tend to abandon exercise altogether. Walking is the most injury-free exercise of all. No other exercise can have that statement made about it.

3. *Exercise must always be accessible.* Sustaining an exercise program under optimum conditions is difficult for the majority of people. If the chosen exercise is not readily available or takes an inordinate amount of time and effort to get to, it is easy to find reasons not to do it once the initial flush of exercise fever wears off.

4. *It must be free.* The people who need exercise the most are at the lower socioeconomic levels. Just getting them up and moving at all is an enormous challenge. If they had to *pay* for an exercise, it would be an even greater challenge. Besides, most of them couldn't afford it. Even if you can afford to pay for exercise, why pay for something if you don't have to? Everyone likes bargains, and it doesn't cost anything to walk.

5. *Exercise should involve the major muscle groups of the upper and lower body (preferably simultaneously) in a nonimpact, dynamic, rhythmic action that will permit the exerciser to achieve an aerobic-training effect.* I have discussed this characteristic with a number of exercise physiologists and doctors. They all agree that it describes what an ideal exercise should consist of. Not everybody will exercise to the aerobic level, but the option to do so should be available.

6. *It should be possible to perform exercise at low-, moderate-, and high-intensity levels.* This range of options in a single exercise permits the most sedentary and/or overweight person to start and continue in the same exercise up to a high level of fitness. I am not suggesting that you abandon any other exercise you like or are doing, or that walking is the *only* exercise worth doing. If you are

just starting an exercise program, however, and are uncertain about which exercise gives you the best all-around weight-control and cardiovascular benefit for your time invested, then you don't have to look any further than exercise walking—it is the complete exercise. As a matter of fact, walking gives you an exercise dimension that no other exercise can give you, and it is unique to walking.

THE SPECIFICITY PRINCIPLE

In my walking clinics, when I ask how many people have ever heard of the *specificity principle of exercise*, I can conservatively say that it is fewer than 2 or 3 out of 100. I found the specificity principle while researching my first book and have had considerable experience with it since. Among exercise physiologists, it is widely known, but the general public has little awareness of it.

This principle is as important in helping you choose an exercise as any of the previously mentioned criteria. In some ways, it is the most important. And it is less intimidating than it sounds. My reference book *Exercise Physiology* explains it in detail.

Here is an example you will readily understand. If you were a champion swimmer in top physical condition, you could not get out of the pool and automatically be a champion runner. Conversely, an Olympic runner can't jump in the pool and be an Olympic swimmer. The training and conditioning necessary to make the muscles fire and perform in one sport are not transferable to another sport. The training effect is sport *specific*—thus, the specificity principle.

As *Exercise Physiology* explains, "Development of aerobic fitness for swimming, bicycling, or running is most effectively achieved when the exerciser trains the specific muscles involved in the desired performance." It concludes, *"Specific exercise elicits specific adaptations creating specific training effects"* (emphasis in original). To test this, the textbook cites a study of 15 men who swam one hour a day, three days a week for ten weeks. The authors expected some aerobic transferability to running, but, when they tested the men running on a treadmill, they found "no effect."

If you are reasonably fit in one sport or exercise but tire quickly in another, *Exercise Physiology* explains, "It is reasonable to advise that in training for specific aerobic activities like cycling, swimming, rowing, or running . . . little improvement is noted when aerobic capacity is measured by a dissimilar exercise. . . . Thus, one can appreciate how difficult it is to be in 'good shape' for diverse forms of exercise." When I read that last sentence six years ago, I wondered why in the world we approach physical exercise any differently than we do mental exercise.

Everyone knows that if you are going to be a lawyer you study law, not basket weaving and applied pottery. If you are going to be an accountant, you study accounting, not first aid and canoeing. We all agree that we put the knowledge into our brain that we intend to take out and use. This raises the question, Why exercise from the neck down any differently than from the neck up?

Doesn't it follow that the exercise we put into our bodies should, like what we put into our minds, be something that has a residual value that we will use every day? *The only physical activity that we use every day is our walking gait.* From the time we crawl out of bed in the morning until we crawl back in at night, walking is our primary gait of locomotion. It has been since Lucy and before, and it will continue to be as long as the human biped exists.

In the course of the day, we substitute automobiles, riding mowers, farm tractors, or whatever mechanical device we need at the time for our walking gait. Even so, walking's role in our lives cannot be replaced entirely. For example, you walk from the house to your car, drive to work, park the car, and walk to your workplace. In the course of your workday, you walk from place to place. After work, you reverse the process. Everything we do is ultimately interspersed with walking. Our problem is that, in our overmechanized world, we have reduced walking's role in our lives to such an extent that it leads to our physical detriment.

Based on the specificity principle, doesn't common sense dictate that *walking should be the foundation exercise for everyone*? Why spend 30 minutes a day on a rowing machine, for instance, knowing that when you get off it you won't be able to walk any better? How much rowing will you be doing during the rest of the day? Proponents of rowing will argue, and rightly so, that it will elevate your heart rate for an aerobic-training effect and burn calories. As a walking proponent, I will tell you that by walking you can also get an aerobic workout, burn as many calories as a rower (or more), *and* you will have enhanced your walking gait so you can function better through the rest of your day. Why exercise 30 minutes one way for a half a loaf when you can get the whole loaf in the same 30 minutes?

WALKING COMPARED
WITH OTHER EXERCISES

With the addition of the specificity principle, we now have *seven criteria* for the ideal lifetime exercise. Armed with them, let's compare walking with a wide range of exercises and exercise equipment. I have read so much about the virtues of all exercise that I have become a 64-year-old cynic. Much of what is recommended is served up to us without regard for the reality of what normal people will or won't do and sometimes without regard for whether it is even possible to do. This last point is one of my pet peeves.

Cross-Country Skiing

I get heartburn every time I read that "cross-country skiing is the number-one aerobic exercise because it uses the major muscles in the upper and lower body." The nonsense in this is that cross-country skiing is hardly more than a *theoretical* exercise for 95 percent of the population. Carol and I have cross-country skis, poles, and boots in the basement and haven't had them on in four years! Not enough snow. How about where you live? How many days a year could you possibly cross-country ski?

Even people who live in the northern tier states, where they have heavy winter snows, cannot cross-country ski year-round. Furthermore, the high aerobic capacity attributed to cross-country skiing was taken from some world-class elite athletes who had trained with duration and intensity beyond the reach of 99.99 percent of the rest of us. Cross-country skiing is a fun recreational exercise, and, if you get a chance, try it. You will find, as I did, however, that, if you poke along slowly, your heart rate doesn't go up. Cross-country skiing is no different from any other aerobic exercise—it takes *intensity* to get a high fitness level. It also takes snow, and walking doesn't.

Swimming

If you are a good swimmer and you like to swim, there isn't anything I could say that would change your mind about swimming. And I wouldn't try if I could. Instead, I would suggest that you work in some walking to supplement your swimming. We are terrestrial animals, not amphibians, and anything you can do to condition your walking gait contributes to your ability to function on land. Remember, when you climb out of the pool, you will walk the rest of the day.

In addition, swimming is not the aid to overweight people it was once thought to be. *Runner's World* magazine cited a study from the University of Missouri that compared the effects of exercise and diet on weight loss in four groups of regular, but slightly overweight, exercisers for a ten-week period. One group ran and dieted; another ran without dieting; a third group swam and dieted; and a fourth swam without dieting.

Randall Smith, clinical assistant professor of physical therapy and principal researcher, said, "We noticed that swimmers are a lot hungrier than runners after workouts." Smith believes that the difference in appetite stems from the hypothalamus, the part of the brain that regulates temperature and appetite. Because water conducts heat away from the body more effectively than air, a swimmer's body temperature remains lower during a workout than a runner's. Smith believes an increased temperature of the hypothalamus is a "turn off" of the desire to eat.

Naturally, *Runner's World* was delighted to report on this study and reminded its readers, "If losing weight is your goal, stick with running." I will remind you, if losing weight *without injury* is your goal, stick to walking—especially aerobic walking. Your hypothalamus doesn't know (or care) whether you walk or run, but either activity deadens your appetite better than swimming.

Swimming has a couple of other drawbacks compared with walking. The freestyle or front crawl, the most popular stroke, utilizes arm pull for as much as 80 percent of the forward motion. The major muscle groups are in your legs, so not only are they not getting enough work but they also aren't working against gravity (as in walking) because they are aided by the buoyancy of the water. Exercising against gravity is recommended for prevention of osteoporosis.

Swimming doesn't score very well against walking on the seven exercise criteria, but, for those who enjoy a good swim, it provides excellent variety when *coupled* with walking.

Outdoor Cycling

Outdoor cycling must be divided into two categories—exercise cycling and recreational cycling. The difference between the two involves speed. To achieve an aerobic fitness level from exercise cycling, according to Dr. Kenneth Cooper, in his book *The Aerobics Program for Total Well-being*, a cycling speed of slightly greater than 15 miles per hour is the optimum rate for a good training effect. He also says, "Generally speaking, speeds of less than 10 miles-per-hour are worth very little from an aerobic standpoint."

Cycling for significant caloric expenditure and aerobic fitness is difficult because of intersections and the problems of traffic in general. There are very few places one can cycle nonstop at speeds greater than 15 miles per hour for 20 minutes or longer. For an aerobic workout, the heart rate should be maintained in the training range for 20 minutes. Stopping, starting, and coasting cause the heart rate to fluctuate.

Consider also that the cyclist primarily uses the quads and very few other major muscle groups. If you've peddled up a hill, you know that the front of your thighs seem to do all the work. When peddling on the flat, the cyclist is sitting on his buttocks—the largest muscle group in the body. All the upper body and its major muscle groups are hunched over the handlebars, totally inactive. Cycling injuries don't come cheap either. A fall at 15 miles per hour can mean broken bones.

Recreational cycling, by contrast, can be used as a complement to a basic aerobic walking program. It is fun and can be done at a leisurely, safe speed as light exercise. Out on my country walking course, there are several husbands and wives who enjoy a leisurely ride on their tandem bikes. I enjoy a good bicycle ride now and then, but my main exercise is walking. Yours should be too.

Racquet Sports

Tennis, racquetball, squash, and badminton are all great games. I was a squash addict until my knee gave out. Some level of fitness can be maintained if the players are competent enough to keep ball (or shuttlecock) in play at an intense level. A hot squash game is a good workout, as are the other racquet sports. But a game such as tennis doubles is not consistently active enough to keep the heart rate elevated. I view racquet sports as fun, recreational activities. They are made even better by a high-intensity aerobic walking program. If you can walk 3 miles in 36 minutes or less, you will have more stamina and less leg fatigue, so you can enjoy your favorite racquet sport even more.

Aerobics and Aerobic Dancing

High-impact aerobics are out and low-impact aerobics are in, say the experts. Aerobic routines come and go, as do the participants. The dropout rate for an average aerobics dance class is about 75 percent. If you are a woman reader of this book, chances are you have tried an aerobics class at least once. Ninety percent of aerobics classes are composed of women.

The death knell for high-impact aerobics was sounded as far back as June 30, 1986, in a full-page story in *Time* magazine. It reported, "A recent survey of 1,200 students found that 43 percent had suffered injuries; among 58 teachers, the figure was an astonishing 76 percent." The injury rate should not be a surprise. As *Time* stated, "An aerobics dancer lands with a force equal to three times her weight." In the article, Peter Francis, a biomechanics researcher at San Diego State University, using slow-motion tapes, observed, "You see a rippling of the skin which is indicative of the shock wave traveling up the body." This high injury rate among participants and teachers spawned low-impact aerobics.

Exercise physiologist Dr. Michael O'Shea explained the difference between high-impact and low-impact aerobics in answer to a reader's question in the October 14, 1990, issue of *Parade* magazine. He said, "The traditional type of aerobic dance has been high-impact aerobics (HIA) which consists of jumping-type activities. . . . Over the past few years HIA has been associated with high injury rates. Shin splints, stress fractures, and tendinitis are common." If those kinds of injuries are "common," is it any mystery why high-impact aerobics is dead?

In an attempt to avoid injuries, aerobic dance instructors have started teaching low-impact aerobics (LIA). Dr. O'Shea said, "LIA is described as maintaining one foot on the floor while performing large upper body movements with wide ranges of motion. . . . To increase intensity, the degree of difficulty of steps, cadence, and amount of work done by the arms versus the legs are varied."

It appears that low-impact aerobics is not injury free either. According to Dr. O'Shea, it has been associated with hyperextension injuries of the shoulder. In addition, exaggerated movements place stress on the knees, ankles, and lower back. The Institute for Aerobics Research, in its January 1988 publication, reported, "Knee injury can stem from the lateral and lunging movements that are usually part of low-impact aerobics routines." The effectiveness of low-impact aerobics is also suspect because it takes a tremendous amount of *unnatural* lunging about to get the heart rate up and keep it there for 20 minutes or longer.

The *Rodale Report*, published by Rodale Press, cited a Ball State University study in which sedentary men and women showed *no* (emphasis in original) improvement in fitness after participating in a 1-hour low-impact aerobics class for 14 weeks. Furthermore, people taking high-impact aerobics classes averaged a 5 percent *loss* in aerobic fitness after switching to low-impact classes.

I have great difficulty suppressing my cynicism about low-impact aerobics as an exercise that makes any sense at all. To me, low-impact aerobics is like trying to reinvent the wheel. Why is everybody trying to create an exercise better than walking? It can't be done.

Furthermore, neither high- nor low-impact aerobics produces *usable* fitness. The arbitrary moves and dance routines may (or may not) elevate your heart rate, but the all-important consideration is the specificity principle. Both aerobics routines fail it miserably. The fitness acquired in these kinds of programs is not transferable to the walking gait. I have some firsthand experience with those who have learned this.

Sue White, a certified aerobics instructor and former Physical Director at the St. Joseph YMCA (now with the YMCA in Ft. Worth, Texas), could take a group of women through a high- or low-impact routine for a fast 30 minutes and have them crying for mercy. Sue is a fine aerobics instructor and highly motivational. She was also in top physical condition—or so she thought. I did some aerobic walking clinics at the St. Joseph Y and got Sue interested. She took a few lessons and picked it up quickly. Then things started to happen.

As Sue got to the 13-minute-mile level, she hit the wall. Her buttocks were sore, her shins were sore, her thighs were heavy, and she was frustrated. All her aerobic bouncing around did not transfer to her walking gait. She had to retrain her leg muscles in their walking mode, then teach them to fire faster in that sequence. She couldn't believe that, as fit as she was, she couldn't do something as seemingly simple as walk fast.

You have to know Sue White to know it wouldn't all end for

her at a 13-minute mile. Within 45 days, she was at the 12-minute mile and shooting for 11. Here's the payoff. Now that Sue is an accomplished aerobic walker, she laughs and admits that she hardly breaks a sweat in her aerobics classes. The high-intensity walking gave her a far greater fitness than all the aerobics routines she was teaching. Sue also admits that she is less tired at the end of the day, because her normal daily walking is almost effortless.

I can recall many other examples, but the one I remember and enjoy the most involves my wife, Carol, and some young aerobics instructors, Las Vegas dancers, and models. In January 1990, NaturalSport hired a Hollywood production company to make a TV commercial about its new Aerobic Walker shoe. The advertising agency decided to show a group of young women walkers walking down a scenic rural road as part of the commercial.

The agency's location manager felt that the Valley of Fire State Park near Lake Mead (about 40 miles outside Las Vegas) had the right look. It is an area of huge red rock formations jutting out of the desert floor.

My assignment, as the walking consultant for NaturalSport, was to meet with a modeling agency to pick out about twenty young, attractive women and teach them aerobic walking so they could be in the commercial. The modeling agency rented an aerobics dance studio. I interviewed the candidates one at a time and asked each to walk back and forth—in her natural manner but at a very brisk pace. This helped me cull out the bouncers and those who had walking peculiarities, such as tracking wide.

I found twenty women I felt would make good aerobic walkers. A few were full-time models. Most were part-time models and Las Vegas dancers, and four were part-time models and *full-time aerobics instructors* at big Las Vegas fitness centers. The aerobics instructors looked terrifically fit in their iridescent tights, matching headbands, and leg warmers. They all had flat tummies and waists about as big around as a small skillet. I specifically asked them if they had ever done any really fast walking for an aerobic workout. They gave this gray-haired guy a look as if I were from another planet. I knew then I was going to have some fun.

After the interviews, I gave a clinic on the aerobic-walking technique. In about an hour all the women looked pretty good, but the dancers really looked great. They had more natural hip rotation than the others and were fluid and rhythmic. They picked up the bent-arm swing quickly, and one remarked, "This is like a dance strut we do in one of our numbers." I sent them home to practice the technique and see if they could put a little speed with it. I was hoping they would all hold up physically when asked to walk short, fast spurts for the TV cameras.

The models were bused out to the Valley of Fire the next morning, and shooting started at 7:45. The last shot was taken at 5:30 P.M. There was a lot of waiting for the camera crew to get set for different shots, so the women were not walking all of that time. My guess is they walked a total of 4 or 5 miles in ⅛-mile spurts at about a 12-minute-mile pace.

The early enthusiasm started to fade by noon. Some were already complaining about their buttocks, their quads, and their shins. By 2:00 P.M. all were making trips to the wardrobe trailer for Tylenol and Advil. That ran out at 4:00 P.M., and we still had an hour and a half to go. When the director finally said, "Cut, that's it—thank you, everybody," they were a bedraggled, relieved bunch. I purposely checked the aerobics instructors to see how they felt. Everyone was sore and dead tired. All admitted they didn't think walking could be that much of a workout.

I mentioned at the beginning that this involved my wife. Carol was on the trip with me, and at dinner the night before the TV shoot Chris, the assistant director, asked her if she was a walker also. I told him she is a tough walker and no one in the commercial would be able to stay with her. Chris told Carol to report to the wardrobe trailer the next morning and he would put her in the commercial.

At the end of the day, Carol filled me in on some of the comments the walkers around her were making in mid- to late afternoon: things like "I can't last another minute of this," "I'll never take another assignment like this," "I think my shins are on fire." Some were registering their discomfort in words that would make a longshoreman blush. Carol and I had a good laugh out of it.

There is no moral to this story, but there *is* a strong lesson in exercise physiology. If you go to an aerobics class—and about 15 to 20 million women a year do—you are not getting as physically fit as if you spent the same amount of time walking at the *intensity* you do your aerobics class. By that I mean that if you have your heart in your aerobic-training range in aerobics class, then all you have to do is walk fast enough to reach your aerobic heart-rate range. Equally important, the specificity principle guarantees that by walking you will have a *usable* physical fitness that contributes to your ability to function in the rest of your daily activities.

Bench-Step Aerobics

The newest exercise craze as this is being written is bench-step aerobics. Fitness publications are jumping on it to tell people what great physical fitness benefits they can get if they step up and down real fast on a bench that is between 6 and 12 inches high. There's more good news. If you swing hand weights around while you're stepping, your fitness is doubled. Gimme a break! No wonder people don't want to exercise.

If you saw your cocker spaniel jumping off and onto the footstool, you would probably wonder out loud, "What's that crazy dog doing?" If you start doing bench-step aerobics and your cocker gives you a funny look, guess what's going through *his* mind. Do both of you a favor and take the dog for a long walk.

Exercise Equipment

Using the seven criteria for a lifetime exercise (with emphasis on the specificity principle), when compared with walking, nothing fails more miserably than exercise equipment. If you have bought a piece and it is gathering dust in the garage, you already know that.

I find many people are highly skeptical that something as basic as walking can be as effective for fitness as a piece of exercise equipment. There seems to be a pervasive belief that some unique physiological alchemy causes fitness to flow into the body from the machine. Don't be hoodwinked. All any exercise equipment does is provide a *mechanical resistance* against which to work your muscles. Read that again, because when you buy exercise equipment you pay a fancy price for mechanical resistance while the best resistance of all, gravity, is free. In truth, most exercise equipment is a waste of money. All kinds of devices designed for you to push, pull, and pedal are being marketed with slick ad campaigns promising cardiovascular and aerobic benefits and better health. If you are not careful, you will part with several hundred to several thousand dollars before finding out not only that most of these contraptions aren't "fun" but also that the boredom of them turns your mind to mush.

The extent to which this industry has grown and the amount of money it is draining from people are astounding. *USA Today* in December 1990 reported the total 1990 sales of exercise equipment would come in at $2 billion!

The November 11, 1990, *Denver Post* noted that the people who make home exercise equipment are starting to get nervous. It posed the question "And if more machines end up in closets will fewer new ones be sold?" A few paragraphs later, "Others in the industry fear that the boom will end as buyers consign their machines to the closet." Architects and home builders should take note and start building bigger closets.

Exercise Cycles

No exercise equipment is more highly promoted and oversold than stationary exercise cycles. The December 1990 *USA Today* article reported, "The stationary bike remains the leading machine—this year 40 million people are expected to ride one, more than half of them at home." My question is, How many times will they ride one—and at what intensity?

I don't like to do it, but sometimes to sell one idea you have to *unsell* another. In the interest of getting you into an exercise-walking program and at the same time save you almost $2,000, let's compare walking with a popular exercise cycle sold in the United States.

An unsolicited brochure for this well-known and widely available exercise cycle came in my mail one day. In it the manufacturer stated, "Stationary bicycling is easy, fun, and burns more calories than any other form of exercise." I have tried this particular unit as well as several similar types, and I can assure you that they aren't "fun" unless you are a masochist. Furthermore, the claim that they burn more calories than other forms of exercise is totally false. The company also claimed that you could get *all* the exercise you need on its cycle in just "12 minutes a day." That is also untrue. All you will get is 12 minutes of mind-numbing exercise.

The friendly price of this computerized exercise cycle is a whopping $1,675. At 1991 prices, you can buy a top-of-the-line exercise-walking shoe for about $70. If you took the $1,675 price of the stationary exercise cycle and divided it by $70, you could buy 24 pairs of shoes. And if you were a pretty aggressive walker and wore out 4 pairs of shoes a year, you would be able to buy exercise-walking shoes for the next 6 years. On your next long walk, think how lucky you are physically and financially to be walking instead of pedaling your way to nowhere.

There is a variation of an exercise cycle called a recumbent cycle. This rig has you leaning back in a chairlike seat while pedaling a flywheel out in front of you. The $699 model I checked out claims that it "makes stress-free exercise a breeze." Of course, the purpose of exercise is to *stress* your physiological system to some extent. You will get out of any "stress-free exercise" exactly what you put into it—not much. The ad for this unit shows an attractive young woman in the seat, fully made up, not a hair out of place, and not a bead of sweat in sight, reading *The Wall Street Journal.* If she is physically "stress free," she is also probably fitness free.

Stair Climbers

The newest form of exercise equipment insanity is stair climbers. If you've gotten tired of cycling to nowhere and rowing to nowhere, you can now climb to nowhere.

In a June 1990 article entitled "Stair Machines: The Truth About This Fitness Fad," *The Physician and Sportsmedicine* stated, "There's nothing magical about the latest fitness craze." As the article pointed out, the obvious alternative to spending money on a stair climber is "Just take the stairs."

If it were that simple, I would leave it there, but it is not. Exercise machines such as stair climbers give the impression that they can produce some magical fitness results and caloric expenditure in a very short time that exercise walking cannot. I know quite a few walkers who spend some of their exercise time on these contraptions in the belief that they are getting concentrated results that would have required a longer time to achieve by walking. Quoting a director of sports sciences at a Denver Health Club, *The Physician and Sportsmedicine* said, "Many health club members seek exercises that expend a lot of energy in a short time."

The magazine also pointed out that today's fitness consumers want equipment with flashy computer screens that blink back physiological data (calorie burn, heart rate, and so on). The health club director said his clients will *wait* for a stair climber that has those features rather than use a noncomputerized device. But the accuracy of computerized stair machines is questioned by Bob Goldman, D.O., director of research at the High Technology Fitness Research Institute in Chicago, a nonprofit organization that tests exercise equipment. He points out, for example, that leaning on the armrests of a stair machine transfers less weight to the pedals and results in the computer's overestimation of calorie expenditure. Everybody I have ever seen using a stair climber was holding or leaning on the armrests; in fact, the advertising pictures show that position.

More important, stair machines are programmed on the basis of the energy required to climb *actual stairs*. Because of the biomechanical differences between climbing a real stationary stair and using a stair-climbing device that gives way with foot pressure, Dr. James Rippe of the University of Massachusetts says, "I have serious reservations as to whether those numbers have meaning."

The exercise equipment business is like Topsy, "it just growed!" Unfortunately, there is no government regulation to make sure these contraptions can deliver what they claim. Without regulations to guarantee the accuracy of computerized exercise results, the equipment manufacturers have free rein to overstate what their devices actually do without regard to the *intensity* and *duration* required to achieve those results. Meanwhile, people will continue to stand in line to climb to nowhere in order to have a computer give them caloric expenditure numbers that may be overstated. Sadly, these same people do not believe a good hard walk will give them better, *usable*, all-around fitness than some piece of exercise equipment will.

The top criteria for a lifetime exercise are that it be natural, not boring, and *reasonably* enjoyable. Other than walking, only jogging is natural, but many people find it boring and few find it enjoyable. The rest of the exercises and exercise equipment simply will *not* be done for a lifetime by the general public. Only walking meets all seven criteria for a lifetime exercise. If the professionals in the exercise movement would start recommending walking to everyone as the *primary exercise*, more people would start to exercise regularly.

Treadmills are Best

I do not own any exercise equipment. However, if I lived in a city where traffic and air pollution forced me to exercise inside, or walking outside was not safe, or the weather was too hot, too cold, or too rainy much of the year, I would buy a treadmill. This is the only piece of exercise equipment that permits you to do the natural exercise of walking and complies with the specificity principle. Walking on a treadmill yields fitness that is transferable to normal daily walking. No other exercise equipment can say that.

Treadmill walking permits you to use the same walking muscles you use when exercise walking on pavement. There is some difference in foot reaction at toe-off on a treadmill, because you are pushing against a surface that is moving in the direction opposite from the way you are walking. But this different feel is only noticeable at an accelerated pace (about a 14-minute mile or faster), and you will probably adapt to the firm surface in less than a mile. It is not a problem.

Treadmills are not cheap; unless you need one for the reasons I have given and are convinced you will use it, save your money. Based on 1991 prices, a good treadmill would cost about $2,000 to $2,500. There are cheaper ones on the market, but they lack adequate horsepower and durability. Buy a good one, or you will waste your money.

Here are six features that a treadmill should have:

1. A *minimum* of 1.5 horsepower, preferably 2.0 horsepower or better. The heavy-duty motor should be quiet.

2. Variable elevation, electronically controlled.

3. Variable speed, up to 8 miles per hour.

4. Ample, sturdy rollers and high-quality padded tread belt for a smooth walking surface. You should not feel *individual* rollers during foot contact with the belt.

5. A walking deck *at least* 4 feet long to accommodate a long stride length.

6. Easy-access controls: on-off switch, elevation button, and variable-speed button.

Those are the basics and all you actually need. Some companies make a deluxe model; for about $1,500 more you can get the computerized panel, with all the bells and whistles and blinking lights. I suggest you buy the basic, heavy-duty unit.

There is one feature on the computerized panel that is worth having: the heart-rate monitor, which gives you your exercise heart rate so you can tell whether you are walking too fast or not fast enough. For a fraction of the cost, though, you can buy one of these separately (see Chapter 11); then, if you exercise walk else-where, you can take it with you.

Here are six tips on how to walk on a treadmill:

- Straddle the belt with each foot on the stationary outside deck and start at a strolling pace of 20 minutes per mile *or less* (3 miles per hour, if that is the calibration used).
- When the belt is moving smoothly, step on and walk at that pace until you establish the rhythm of your walk and feel totally relaxed and coordinated.
- Increase the belt speed gradually over several minutes, always making sure you have your posture, technique, and rhythm in sync.
- Try to increase heart rate with walking speed rather than by elevating the treadmill. Walk fast with the treadmill flat or ele-vated no more than a few degrees to get your heart rate up.

  You can also elevate the treadmill to the level of a gradual hill and elevate your heart rate by walking much slower. I believe it is better to reach your aerobic-training range using a faster walk-ing pace on a nearly flat surface because this way you are getting your leg muscles to fire faster. This method gives you the residual ability to walk faster and with less effort in your normal daily walking. There may be days, however, when you don't want to work your legs so hard. By elevating the treadmill to a level where you can maintain erect posture and rhythm, you can hit your training range walking much more slowly. Experiment to find the elevation that feels right for you. Try not to elevate the treadmill any more than necessary, however, so that you can maintain correct posture.

- Do not hold the handrails. If you have to hold the handrails to keep your balance, you have the treadmill going too fast relative to your walking ability. You don't hold on to anything walking at your top pace down a road, so why should it be different on a treadmill? Let your arms swing freely.

  Walkers at the brisk and particularly the aerobic bent-arm swing pace must have a good loose arm swing to counterbalance their lower-body rotations. Just as important, using the vigorous arm swing involves six major muscle groups in the upper body that would be inactive if you were holding the handrails. Never settle for half a loaf of exercise when you can get it all in the same amount of time.

- Don't use hand weights on a treadmill or *ever* in an exercise-walking program. (More about them in Chapter 11.)

Do not be surprised if you can't walk as fast on pavement as you can on a treadmill. The moving belt seems to aid foot turnover from heel plant to toe-off. With the bent-arm swing, it is easier to hit a 12-minute mile on a treadmill than on pavement. Even so, it does not take much pavement walking to catch up with your treadmill-walking proficiency.

If you get your exercise at a fitness center, *remember the specificity principle*. Walk right on by the exercise cycles, rowing machines, and stair climbers, and get your workout on a treadmill.

THE OLD WALKER VERSUS THE YOUNG RUNNER

"The calm confidence of a Christian with four aces" was Mark Twain's description of someone who knew with metaphysical certitude that he or she was in a predictable winning situation. As an admirer of Twain's writings, I had that quote flash through my mind one day in the spring of 1990 when I was on my national tour for NaturalSport walking shoes. I had a late afternoon to kill before an evening walking clinic. Across the boulevard from the Marriott Hotel in downtown Portland, Oregon, is a wide, paved path in a park that runs along the Willamette River for several miles. With the river on one side and the grassy park area on the other, it is a refreshing and mentally stimulating place to walk.

There were a lot of runners and cyclists using the path this day and a few older, slower walkers. It was a gray afternoon with a little nip in the air. I put on my sweats and nylon windbreaker and headed up along the river. I was cruising along at a pretty comfortable pace (about a 12-minute mile) when two young male runners came up beside me. They walked with me for about 20 yards, mimicking my bent-arm swing. We made eye contact, and I could see they were feeling their oats and just clowning around. Finally, the one closest to me said, "Sorry, old man, this is too slow for us, we'll see you around," and they took off running. Five minutes later I saw them stopped up ahead, talking to a couple of female cyclists who were obviously friends.

As I approached, I could see they were watching me and talking about the way I was walking. When I got to them I smiled and said, "I don't think you took off running because I was too slow, I think it was because you can't walk as fast as I can!" They took the bait. One of the guys said, "Aw, come on, walking is for old people. Anybody can do that." I took a fifty-dollar bill out of the money clip I had in my windbreaker and said, "I'll bet you fifty dollars I can beat you walking down to the end of the path in front of the Marriott and back to here." By my calculation that was a bit more than 2 miles. (As a word of caution, it is not wise to carry a lot of money when out walking. However, the bell captain at the hotel assured me that this was a safe area, and I preferred having the money in my pocket to leaving it in the hotel room.)

The one young guy said, "That's a safe bet for you because we don't have fifty dollars." I had suspected that when I made the challenge, and now I had them where I wanted them. I said, "Okay, I'll *give* you this fifty-dollar bill if you can beat me, and if you lose you don't have to give me anything." Now I had the girls on my side, and one said, "Come on, Steve, take him up on it—what have you got to lose—you can beat him." Steve, I found out later, was a 20-year-old college miler with a personal best time of 4 minutes, 9 seconds for the mile. I'm glad I found that out *later* or I might not have waved that fifty-dollar bill at him. He just looked to me like another young runner who didn't know how the specificity principle works with walking.

After considerable cajoling from the girls, Steve decided to take my walking challenge. I said there was only one stipulation: that his weight-bearing leg had to be straight when it passed under him so that he was not using bent knees in a flat-footed run. I showed him what I meant. Steve walked about 20 paces to try it and said, "No problem." We lined up to start. Steve's friend, Brad, stayed back at the finish line. The girls decided to cycle up and back with us to watch the race and to shout encouragement to Steve.

We took off walking, and I could see that Steve's early strategy was to let me set the pace. My mile walk down to them had been just perfect for a warm-up. My walking muscles were ready, my rhythm felt good, and the temperature of about 55 degrees was perfect.

I locked in at an easy 11-minute-mile pace for the first 6 minutes, and Steve stayed right with me. Young, fit legs are hard to tire and at 62 my old legs were spotting him 42 years in age. I kept checking my stopwatch, and when we hit 6 minutes I knew we were more than halfway through the first mile. By now my leg muscles were firing easily, my arm swing was loose, my rhythm was smooth, and my adrenaline was pumping. It was time to turn the heat up a little.

I increased my walking speed to about a 10-minute-mile pace for the rest of the first leg. We had gone about a quarter of a mile at that speed, and Steve was hanging right in there with me. A trickle of doubt started to seep into my mind.

A couple of minutes later, however, my confidence was restored. Not only did I have four aces but I owned the stacked deck. As we made the turn to head back, I glanced over at Steve. He had a bewildered, stricken look. Eyes speak volumes when fatigue shows up. I felt a new surge of adrenaline and confidence and decided it was time to see what this young fellah was made of.

I have never walked in a competitive race in my life. In fact, this day was the most competitive I have ever been. Out on my country walking course, I have timed myself at a 9-minute mile at least a half dozen times and an 8-minute, 47-second mile once. I knew if push came to shove I could do a 9-minute mile, and this was the time to do it. I kicked in the afterburners and took off. Steve was with me for about 40 yards, and then, as he told me later, his coordination was gone, his motor neurons wouldn't fire his leg muscles, his shin muscles were on fire, and he couldn't lift his feet fast enough for each step.

I was rolling now and widened the distance between us with every step. At this point, the only thing at issue was by how far I would beat him. When I reached Brad, Steve was about ⅛ mile behind. Once he saw he was beat, he jogged in to give his legs a *rest*. Steve admitted that he had never experienced fatigue like that from running. The confusing thing to him was that, when he sent a signal from his brain to his legs to move faster, nothing happened. His leg muscles had not been specifically trained in the walking gait to fire that fast over that distance, so when extreme fatigue set in they couldn't respond.

Before I said good-bye to the four young people, the girls parked their bicycles and asked me to show them how to walk that fast. They were both naturals and picked up the bent-arm-swing technique in a few minutes. They were amazed at how fast they could walk. Testing their newfound speed, they walked out about 200 yards and back as fast as they could. By the time they got back, their shins were on fire, and they realized the problem Steve had had in the last mile.

The old dogma that runners are more fit than aerobic walkers or race walkers is as up-to-date as the flat earth doctrine. They are fit as runners only. Their specificity of running does not transfer to walking. It is a sure bet that a walker who can walk 10-minute miles or faster will beat a good runner in a 2- or 3-mile walk if the runner hasn't cross-trained in walking.

There is one major exception to the specificity principle, however, but it is the exact opposite of what most people would guess. I believe it is the most significantly overlooked, underutilized aspect of aerobic exercise and athletic training. Read on.

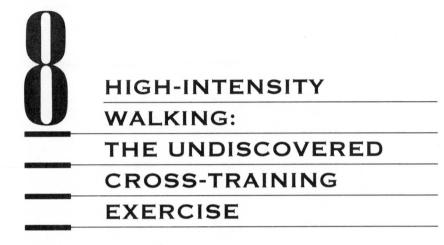

8 HIGH-INTENSITY WALKING: THE UNDISCOVERED CROSS-TRAINING EXERCISE

At 4:05 P.M., I headed east out Countyline Road for my late-afternoon walk. It was Monday, September 10, 1990, a pivotal day during my research for this book. The sun was behind me and slightly to the south. Summer was fading, and the shadows were starting to slant north as early autumn eased into northwest Missouri. I was swept along by an adrenaline rush and euphoric anticipation, and my pace was effortlessly quick. Two unrelated, unexpected events bonded by a common purpose made this day special. It was the kind of happening that makes coincidence seem too simplistic.

The first event was a 10:00 A.M. telephone call from Dr. William Byrnes of the Human Performance Laboratory at the University of Colorado, Boulder. He wanted to share the news of an exciting new development in a major walking study he was conducting for NaturalSport. The second came in the mail at 2:30. To my total surprise, a magazine article by a highly respected runner, writer, and physician reinforced my lingering intuition about high-intensity walking as an athletic cross-training aid.

THE OXYGEN UPTAKE CLUE

In the spring of 1985, when I was researching my first book, *Aerobic Walking*, I had found a graph (Figure 8.1) that was part of a study of the relationship of oxygen intake and velocity of walking and running in competition walkers. The numbers across the bottom of the chart indicate the walker's speed in kilometers per hour. (Since kilometers are not widely used in the United States and are unfamiliar to most, a key number to remember is 8 kilometers, which equals 5 miles per hour, which is the equivalent of 12-minute miles.) I added the circle to the graph to focus your attention on the point where the lines of oxygen utilization between walking and running cross, which is about 8 kilometers per hour. This is called a metabolic intersection, where the energy costs of two activities meet. It was apparent even to my untrained eye that, from about a 12-minute mile on, a walker uses considerably more oxygen than a runner if both maintain the same speed. I find most people don't believe this or understand it. Even though an exercise walker could not achieve the top speeds of these competition walkers, many aerobic walkers walk 12-minute miles or faster. In fact, at the time I found the graph I was routinely walking at a 10- or 11-minute-mile pace on my daily walks.

It was this graph that motivated me to see how high I could elevate my fitness level by high-intensity walking. I had received some instruction on the race-walking technique from Larry Young, the USA's only Olympic race-walking medalist at the current distances. I am not very good at it, and I do not consider myself a race walker. I just get out on the country roads near my home and walk hard, using the bent-arm-swing technique that I described in Chapter 6. I figured, however, that if I could keep walking well beyond that metabolic intersection shown in Figure 8.1, I should develop the fitness of a good runner.

In June of 1985 I went to the Cooper Clinic to have my fitness level tested by Dr. Boyd Lyles. By that time I could walk 7 miles in 70 minutes. The Cooper Clinic has conducted over 100,000 treadmill stress tests and has the largest bank of comparative fitness values in the world. From these tests it has constructed "Definition of Fitness Categories" charts for males and females.

I was 57, and my treadmill time that day was 28 minutes and 32 seconds, which exceeded the highest rating for males *30 and younger*. I had also reduced my body fat composition to only 13 percent. Dr. Lyles was so impressed with my performance that he had the clinic's publications department do an article about me for their monthly periodical. The cover story in that issue was about Tatu, who in 1985 and 1986 was the most valuable professional soccer player in the United States. He'd had his fitness tested on the treadmill a week after I did. My time was 47 seconds *better* than his, and Tatu was *34 years younger*.

I also became curious about something Larry Young had mentioned the previous year when I'd asked him what problems he encountered in training for an Olympic race. Larry said getting highly fit and staying fresh were sometimes difficult. He remembered that, when he tended to get stale in the late stages of training, he would occasionally *run* the last 5 miles of a 10-mile workout at about an 8-minute-mile pace to relax his mind and his legs. Larry said running was less intense mentally and physically than walking at that pace and it seemed to freshen him up. I asked him if he could have run much faster than an 8-minute-mile pace, and he said he was sure he could, but speed was not his reason for running.

This intrigued me. How could an athlete training for a specific event unrelated to running run 5 miles in 40 minutes literally on a whim *without cross-training* and, in fact, do it because it seemed relatively effortless? I felt sure a swimmer, a cyclist, or a rower could not do that. Was this an aberration in the specificity principle? Could distance runners who ran at a 5-minute-mile pace, for instance, switch to a walk and walk at perhaps a 9-minute-mile pace? Was this unique, that a high-intensity walker could transfer his or her aerobic capacity to running, or does the running gait possess a similar reciprocity with walking?

My mind was buzzing with questions. I got the graph in Figure 8.1 out again and drew the dotted lines down to the kilometers-per-hour line from the fastest walking speed and the fastest running speed. It showed that those competitive walkers had walked at a pace of about 6.6-minute miles but also ran at speeds up to 5.4-minute miles. Were they cross-trained? If not, how could they do that without cross-training? How could they achieve a higher oxygen intake walking than running? Isn't running supposed to require more oxygen for a higher aerobic capacity than walking?

The study clearly showed that these competitive walkers were capable of developing oxygen uptakes comparable to those of many

FIGURE 8.1

*Relationships between oxygen consumption and velocity for
walking and running on a treadmill in competition walkers*

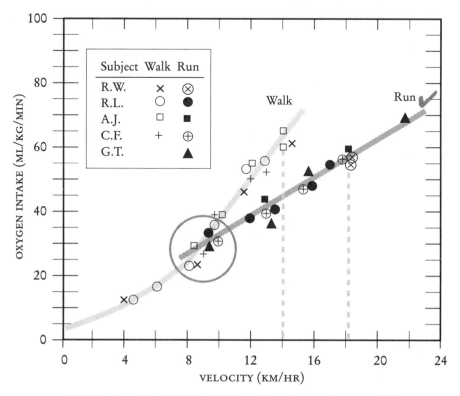

SOURCE: D.R. Menier and L.G.C.E. Pugh, "The relation of oxygen intake and velocity
of walking and running in competition walkers," *J.Physiol.* 197:717, 168.

competitive runners. There seemed to be another subtlety hidden
in the study. These walkers were also able to develop *velocities*
(5.4-minute pace) similar to those of distance runners, apparently
without cross-training. I say apparently because I had no way of
proving they hadn't cross-trained. I could only assume it.

If my assumption was correct, the possibilities of using high-
intensity walking for aerobic athletic conditioning and training
seemed endless. Those unorthodox thoughts were still bouncing
around in the back of my head the day my friend Dolph Bridgewater and I shook hands and I became the walking consultant for

NaturalSport walking shoes. I believed duplicating this study with competitive walkers who were *definitely not cross-trained* was imperative to resolve the question.

THE NATURALSPORT CROSS-TRAINING STUDY

The management team at NaturalSport gave me the green light for a new study. They saw the expanded role high-intensity walking could play in athletic training and realized it would call for a specifically designed high-performance walking shoe. My search for a top exercise physiologist with research experience to conduct the study led me to Dr. William Byrnes of the Department of Kinesiology at the University of Colorado, Boulder. He checked the scientific literature and found that no one had ever tested for such a cross-training effect. Dr. Byrnes enlisted his friend and former college mentor, Dr. Jay T. Kearney, the head of Sports Science at the United States Olympic Training Center (USOTC), to assist in the protocol design and testing. We were on our way.

The study that resulted in Figure 8.1 was conducted in 1968 by D. R. Menier and L. G. C. E. Pugh in the Pyrenees Mountains, at a French Olympic training center. The four competitive walkers in the study were in training for the 1968 Olympics. No runners were tested. Dr. Byrnes's protocol had a clever wrinkle. He felt our study would be more comprehensive if he tested walkers *and* runners who were not cross-trained in the opposite gait. He could then measure the aerobic transferability in both directions. To establish a standard level of athletic competence for the athletes to be tested, he and Dr. Kearney decided to test only competitive walkers who were capable of walking at an 8-minute-mile pace or better for 10 kilometers (6.2 miles). The runners had to be capable of running at a 6-minute-mile pace or better for 10 kilometers. We wanted nationally ranked athletes.

The actual protocol was quite extensive and complex. In simple lay language, however, it boiled down to this. Each participant had to walk on a motorized treadmill at predetermined progressive speeds to reach a heart rate of 170. At that point, the treadmill grade was increased by 2.5 percent every 2 minutes until the subject reached volitional exhaustion. On a separate day the participants would repeat a similar process using the running gait.

For simplicity of recruiting top athletes and conducting the tests in the most convenient location, it was decided to do the physical aspects of the study at the USOTC. This turned out to be the reason for Dr. Byrnes's excited call to me on September 10. The Mexican National Race-walking Team was coming in late September for some physiological testing on the USOTC's sophisticated equipment, and Dr. Kearney had persuaded them to participate in our study.

This was a real coup. The Mexicans are some of the best walkers in the world. Dr. Byrnes was excited because he would now be able to test world-class athletes with exceptional ability who figured to have large aerobic capacities. He and Dr. Kearney had tested the U.S. men's race-walking team in August, and the U.S. women's team was to be tested in November.

To my disappointment, my travel schedule did not permit me to observe the U.S. men's test or the Mexicans'. I was able to attend the women's test, however. Five of the six women walkers who were tested are on both the U.S. race-walking team and the NaturalSport Women's Race-walking Team. When I walked into the USOTC Sports Science Building on November 10, three of our walkers—Lynn Weik, the American road record holder for the 15K and 20K; Teresa Vaill, 1990 and 1991 indoor 3K champion; and Susan Liers, who held several American records in the late 1970s—were lounging about on the floor doing their stretches in preparation for the treadmill tests.

I watched those young women walk to exhaustion one day and run to exhaustion the next. It was like an athletic endurance contest. As each one neared volitional exhaustion, her fellow walkers, Dr. Kearney, Dr. Byrnes, and I joined in to root them on. This was a tough protocol.

On Sunday afternoon, November 11, when all the tests were completed, Dr. Kearney gathered the race walkers and gave them a personalized classroom lecture on some of the subtleties of physical conditioning and how they might develop higher levels of athletic performance through better training regimens. He has a warm, fatherly approach, and our young women walkers were drinking it in.

I have a deep sense of confidence that our Olympic athletes are getting the best technical advice possible from this concerned professional. Dr. Kearney also has a wry sense of humor, and he concluded his session by saying, "Everything I have just told you will work up to a point, but you should all know that the most important decision you or any athlete must make *is choosing the right set of parents,*" and he broke into a broad grin. They understood. Then he added, "Discipline and determination are essential, but, without genetics also, an athlete cannot win the gold." Class dismissed.

All during the testing time, I questioned Dr. Byrnes about when we would test some nationally ranked runners. Drs. Kearney and Byrnes had begged, pleaded, coaxed, and cajoled many runners and running teams of the competency level they needed to take the two treadmill tests. A few agreed to do the running test, but *none would do the walking*! All participants of the study had to be volunteers. None were paid, and all the race walkers had willingly volunteered. I have long suspected that most of the big-name runners are a pampered, idolized, overpaid bunch. Now I was convinced my suspicions were correct, and I was hot!

It was unthinkable in my view that someone of Dr. Kearney's importance and stature at the Olympic level could not persuade a few runners to take a treadmill test for a protocol which might demonstrate an aerobic cross-training effect that could be used by *all* athletes. It was not an unreasonable request. The great irony of this is that, if the aerobic transferability premise was correct, training regimens for runners could be altered to incorporate some high-intensity walking, which could probably reduce running injuries. Runners would ultimately gain far more than walkers.

Dr. Byrnes quickly calmed my fears that the study would be flawed without the runners. He pointed out that the main thrust of the study was to see if high-intensity walking could produce a similar oxygen uptake in the running gait without cross-training. For that we needed walkers—which we had. The runners were not critical to the study.

HUNCH PROVEN CORRECT

On April 19, 1991, Bill Byrnes, Jay Kearney, and I left the Hotel Georgia in Vancouver, Canada, and headed down Howe Street to the Vancouver Trade and Convention Center, where the International Congress on Sports Medicine and Human Performance was being held. They were going to present the results of our study. I helped Bill and Jay post the study abstract and the many charts that were the result of the testing. An abstract is a brief factual summarization.

FIGURE 8.2

*Racewalking and running maximal oxygen uptakes
for United States and Mexican national team members*

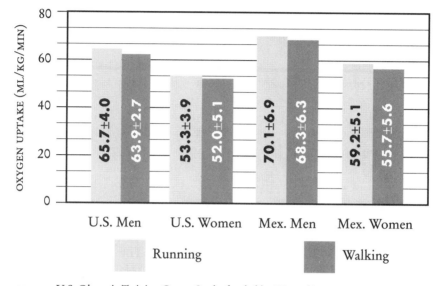

SOURCE: U.S. Olympic Training Center Study, funded by NaturalSport.

The abstract for this study begins: "Fifteen national team race walkers (RW) (9 males and 6 females) from the United States (US) and ten national RW (5 males and 5 females) from Mexico (Mex) agreed to participate in a series of physiological tests." Then followed all the statistical data and procedural explanations. It was the last sentence of the abstract that leaped out at me. It said, *"These athletes are capable of achieving similar VO₂ max values for race walking and running, which indicates a potential cross-training effect."* I kept reading that sentence over and over because I believed it threw open the door for high-intensity walking to be utilized as a new approach to athletic training. My premise had at last moved from speculation to hard data.

Bill posted a graph (Figure 8.2) that illustrated the *average* race-walking and running maximal oxygen uptakes for U.S. and Mexican national team members. It clearly shows that all these athletes were able to achieve similar VO₂ max values in both the running and walking gait *without cross-training*!

For the average person reading this book, the term *maximal oxygen uptake* doesn't have much meaning. It is an important measurement, however, used by exercise physiologists to determine the limit of oxygen utilization attainable by an athlete (or individual) based on his or her level of aerobic fitness. The Menier and Pugh study used the term *oxygen intake*, which means the same thing.

The highest average numbers ever achieved in oxygen uptake were by some very elite, highly trained cross-country skiers who were able to reach the mid-80s. According to Jay Kearney, a "handful of elite runners may hit the low 80s," but most elite runners will test in the upper 70s. Very good nationally ranked runners will test in the low 70s or upper 60s. The averages shown here are excellent because they were achieved in *both* the walking and running gait without the benefit of cross-training. One male Mexican walker actually had an oxygen uptake of 77 walking and 78 running. That is a phenomenal performance, and, as Jay said several times, "Those Mexicans have *big engines!*"

By "big engines" Jay meant their *hearts*. The Mexican men's hearts in particular had enormous capacities to pump huge volumes of blood at relatively few beats per minute for the work they were doing. Figure 8.3 shows the Mexican men's "engines" compared with the Americans' during the walking part of the protocol. At every measured velocity across the bottom of the chart, their hearts were beating considerably *less* than the American men's. This indicates that the Mexicans can carry their speed over a great distance with less fatigue. In other words, they will win the race.

There is an interesting parallel between this study and the one in 1968. Menier and Pugh made a specific notation that an internationally ranked marathon runner serving as a control in their study *"had a VO$_2$ max of 70 ml/Kg/min—a surprisingly high value considering the altitude"* (see check mark on the right-hand side in Figure 8.1). That study was conducted at 5,940 feet. The elevation of Colorado Springs is *6,035 feet,* so the oxygen uptakes generated in that rarefied atmosphere by all of the walkers are indeed impressive.

As I studied the graph, I was groping for a way to explain to readers of this book how those numbers might relate to athletes in other sports. In sports, for instance, that we all watch and whose participants we assume to be highly fit and superbly conditioned. As an Ohio State University graduate, I am naturally a football

FIGURE 8.3

A comparison of the heart rate responses during racewalking for the male members of the United States and Mexican national teams between 7.0 and 8.5 mph

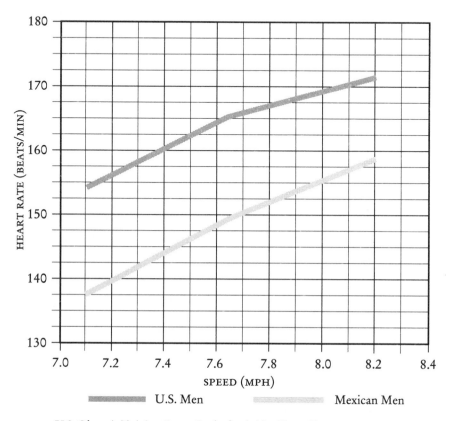

SPEED (MPH)

▬▬▬▬ U.S. Men   ▬▬▬▬ Mexican Men

SOURCE: U.S. Olympic Training Center Study, funded by NaturalSport.

fan, so I asked Jay if the oxygen uptake of around 70 milliliters per kilogram per minute would normally be duplicated by football players. In mock dismay he said, "Oh, Casey! If you collected *all* of the NCAA Division One football players who have an oxygen uptake above seventy, you could invite them over for dinner tonight and not be in trouble with Carol." I assumed that would be true for linemen and linebackers, but I asked if it would also be true for the great running backs.

There was a confident smile on Jay's face as he cranked the

certainty of his answer up a notch. He said, "That would definitely be true for running backs also. I expect you could go to the Kansas City airport [the one I use] and pick them all up in your car." Bill Byrnes broke into a wide grin and added, "I have a hunch you won't even have to go to the Kansas City airport." Both laughed as Jay concurred, "Casey, I have a feeling you're going to have a *very small party.*" If top college football running backs do not have that level of oxygen uptake, what would basketball players, baseball players, tennis players, or hockey players have?

The walking gait has been considered a "moderate activity" and has not been tested at high-intensity levels. Although the 1968 study by Menier and Pugh established a high oxygen uptake for Olympic-level walkers, no one picked up on the fact that these athletes actually had a *double-gaited fitness* and could transfer their walking fitness to the running gait. The study by Drs. Byrnes and Kearney has clearly demonstrated again that an Olympic-caliber race walker can transfer a high aerobic fitness level to running without cross-training. The only question remaining then is, Would high-intensity walking performed at levels considerably *less* than Olympic-caliber race walking have a trickle-down effect? Would it produce the fitness and aerobic capacity needed by NCAA Division 1 football players, NFL football players, basketball players, baseball players, tennis players, and hockey players? I am confident it would.

MY PERSONAL EXPERIMENT

There was one nagging loose end about all of this still in the back of my mind that had to be resolved. I wanted to know if I could transfer *my* fitness level from walking back to running. I had procrastinated for several years on trying to find out because I feared doing irreparable harm to my fragile right knee.

In February 1984, that knee had turned to mush from running. The cartilage on the medial side was gone, and the knee was constantly swollen. My orthopedic doctor finally said, "Your running days are over!" I have not run ten steps since. On November 1, 1990, I had my annual physical at the Cooper Clinic, and I tested superior on the treadmill for a 50-year-old and excellent for a 30-year-old and younger. Not as good as my 1985 treadmill test, but I had reduced my walking frequency, duration, and intensity since an arthroscopic knee operation in 1987 to prolong the time before I might have to have an artificial replacement for my arthritic right knee.

On November 2, the day after my physical, I decided it was time to see if I could run as fast as or faster than I walk. I was in excellent physical condition, but the thought of running on my arthritic knee had all the appeal of a root canal. I dreaded doing it, but I knew I would never have peace of mind until I did. I believe so strongly in the premise of walking's aerobic transferability to running that, if I didn't experience it personally, it would never seem a reality. To me, it was the difference between reading about an earthquake and standing there while the ground shakes under your feet.

At 10:30 A.M. I started walking down my 2-mile flat course on Riverside Road. I decided I would walk the first mile at a comfortable 12-minute-mile pace to warm up. It was a delightfully cool morning with just the hint of a breeze. The conditions were perfect. At the ½-mile mark I was pretty well warmed up and walking effortlessly at a shade less than a 12-minute-mile pace when a moment of indecision hit me. Here I was within 50 days of my sixty-third birthday, in perfect health, financially secure, enjoying life, and I was about to premeditatedly run, which I'd been warned never to do again.

My commitment was irreversible, however; I wavered only for a moment. At the 1-mile mark I hit my stopwatch and apprehensively started to run for the first time in *six years and seven months.* If my knee held up, I had decided, I would run 2 miles at an easy loping pace. Eight- to 9-minute miles had been my regular pace during my running days.

The first couple of hundred yards seemed strange and fairly effortless, but I quickly realized I didn't have a sense of a running pace anymore. I couldn't tell if I was in a slow jog or running at a respectable speed. I also noticed that I was running with a slight limp. My knee wasn't actually hurting, but I was expecting it to, so I was consciously favoring my right leg. I was running unbalanced, which I knew would contribute to unnecessary fatigue in my good leg, so I got back on an even keel with both legs—for a while.

After half a mile, I was breathing a bit more heavily than when I am in a 10-minute-mile high-intensity walk, but I wasn't short of breath and knew I could go faster if I wanted to. At the ¾-mile mark, I was curious about what my pace was and anxious to finish the first mile. As I hit the orange mile mark I have at the side of the road, I glanced at my stopwatch. It registered 8 minutes, 52 seconds. Piece of cake! I turned and headed back for the second mile.

At the ¼-mile mark, I was starting to feel some pain in the right knee. It wasn't imaginary this time, but it didn't become constant until I had passed the ½-mile mark. By then I was consciously running with a limp but determined to finish. When I hit the mile mark, my stopwatch registered 18 minutes and 6 seconds for the 2 miles. My knee felt as if it were on fire in deep on the medial side, where the cartilage is gone, but I was smiling anyhow. I knew I could have gone faster if the knee had been sound. The results of the study at the USOTC were yet to come, but at that moment my *personal* study had proven my point. Although the scientific community calls what I did "anecdotal," I knew what I did had to be grounded in the walking gait's apparent aberration in the specificity principle. It was not an accidental fluke that at almost 63 years of age and not having run in over six years I could run 2 miles at a 9-minute-mile average. You can't fake that.

Once the momentary euphoria of my accomplishment wore off, I became quite aware of my painful right knee. The 5-minute ride home seemed twice as long as normal. When I hit the house, I downed two aspirin, took a hot shower, and had an ice pack on the knee, all in the space of about 7 minutes. The rest of the day was spent on the couch with the ice pack. By evening the pain had settled down, and there was no swelling. I took two aspirin at bedtime and had a deep sleep of satisfaction. The next morning the knee was a little tender, but after two days of rest I was back out walking with no pain. In this instance, being a guinea pig was well worth it. I had felt the ground shake.

The study at the USOTC probably sheds less light on how high-intensity walking can be converted to a universal form of athletic conditioning than what I did on Riverside Road that November day. The Olympic-class race walkers demonstrated that very high oxygen uptakes can be achieved with very high-intensity walking and then be transferred to the running gait without cross-training. But they did it at a walking speed unattainable by most other athletes.

That's the bad news. The good news is that other athletes don't need those kinds of oxygen uptakes for their athletic conditioning. Only other race walkers, middle- and long-distance runners, and cross-country skiers need oxygen capacity in those ranges. I was able to demonstrate the trickle-down effect of aerobic transferability. My walking intensity in the 10- to 12-minute-mile range was convertible to a 9-minute-mile running pace at the age of 63 —and with a bum knee at that. Imagine what kind of double-gaited aerobic conditioning a young male or female athlete with two good legs could achieve with high-intensity walking.

A RESPECTED RUNNER
SPEAKS UP FOR WALKING

No one hungers more for validity than the solitary contrarian trying to scale a wall of conventional wisdom. Scientific giants like Copernicus and Galileo experienced that hunger when they reasoned that the earth revolves around the sun. Intellectuals and scholars at the great universities of their time rejected such unconventional thinking. In my lonely pursuit to establish walking as a viable cross-training exercise for running and other physical activities that require an elevated aerobic capacity, I had yearned for someone who shared my vision. Not just anyone, but someone who commanded the respect of the entire exercise community. On September 10, 1990, at 2:30 P.M., my yearning was fulfilled beyond all expectations. As I walked down to the road to pick up the mail, I was still levitating with excitement about Bill Byrnes's call. In the mail was the September issue of *The Physician and Sportsmedicine* magazine, which I look forward to each month. It supplies me with interesting articles and up-to-date research on various aspects of exercise.

I dumped the mail on my rolltop desk and settled into my Lincoln rocker to scan the magazine for articles of special interest. On page 31, I found my favorite feature, Dr. George Sheehan's monthly column. The title hit me between the eyes like a kick from a Missouri mule. It read, "Walking: Underrated Training Aid." I devoured the page, then I got my highlight marker out and went through it two more times. Dr. Sheehan speculated on all my premises about using walking as an athletic training aid and even opened up possibilities I had overlooked.

While many readers of this book may not have heard of George Sheehan, anyone who has been a serious runner certainly should have. He is considered the patriarch of the running movement. The permanent title for his column in *The Physician and Sportsmedicine* is "Running Wild." Dr. Sheehan is also the medical editor for *Runner's World* and the author of many books related to running, including *Medical Advice for Runners* and *Running and Being*. Dr. Sheehan is in his early seventies and retired from his medical practice after almost forty years as a cardiologist. At major running events and physical-fitness meetings, Dr. Sheehan is sought after as a speaker. Among hard-core runners, he commands respect bordering on adulation. No one has a better insight into runners' mentality, even how they view walking and walkers. Now in his later years, he occasionally walks as a substitute for his usual runs and freely admits that, while walking, "I come up with as many good ideas as I do on a run."

As a keen observer of his fellow runners, Sheehan noticed their disdain for walkers during one of his walks: "I saw a runner friend approaching me. I raised my hand in greeting but he ran right by without recognizing me." Sheehan now takes note of runners passing when he walks, and rarely do they give him a glance. "Yet if I were running, I know I would get a friendly word, or at least a wave," he said.

I had long suspected that most runners view walking with contempt, but I wasn't aware of the depth of that contempt until Dr. Sheehan wrote in his September 1990 column: "Walkers and walking are of no interest to runners. They regard walking as an entry-level exercise practiced by non-athletes, a low-intensity, non-competitive pursuit that has no place in the exciting world of road racing. . . . I think most runners have the idea that walking has nothing to offer them relative to training for their sport." I am sure Sheehan didn't know how prescient this comment was. Almost ninety days to the day after I read Dr. Sheehan's article, Bill Byrnes informed me that he and Jay Kearney could not get any runners to volunteer for the walking part of the study at the USOTC.

Dr. Sheehan went on to speculate on how wrong the runners might be: "Runners with this attitude may well be ignoring a valuable, perhaps even essential element in their conditioning." Dr. Sheehan's column was based on the way some highly respected coaches had conditioned their athletes at the turn of the century.

He specifically mentioned Harry Andrews, who coached a great runner named Alfie Shrubb. At one time Shrubb held all the world records for distances from 2 to 15 miles. "Many other runners, boxers, and cyclists of the time were followers of the Andrews method," Dr. Sheehan said. The one thing they had in common? *They all spent considerable time walking.*

According to Andrews, it did not matter whether your sport was boxing, fencing, wrestling, rowing, running, javelin, or shot put; walking as a primary exercise was applicable to all. He felt it was nature's first exercise and offered "by far the greatest benefit of any form of training in its results." Andrews's program for his budding runners consisted mostly of walking, interspersed with occasional running. Even as these athletes progressed, Andrews continued a policy of morning and evening walks. Running was limited to the afternoon, and *the time spent walking always exceeded that spent running.*

For those interested only in fitness, Andrews recommended walking; he saw it as a superior way to reduce weight. His instructions were simple: "The best advice I can give is make your own pace—the pace, in fact, that will suit you best. This pace will almost certainly be an average of 4 miles an hour."

Somewhere between 1900, when that sage advice was given, and the 1990s, walking was shunted aside as a useful part of an athlete's training regimen, the philosophy being that the only way to improve speed is to practice speed. That may be true, but any runner's training regimen should include the right amount of "recovery miles." High-intensity walking could play an important role in this phase of training. Many studies have shown that when duration and intensity are increased, the injury rate for runners increases dramatically. This is not true for walkers—at any intensity level.

In an effort to reduce injuries and improve performance, there is a current trend among coaches and runners to use what is known as "cross-training." As Dr. Sheehan pointed out, "Runners are now encouraged to substitute some of their running time with cycling, swimming, or weight lifting." But, he added, "when we think about alternative types of training, we should consider walking, the primary cross-training activity of the early 1900's." Dr. Sheehan concluded, "It is possible that walking will enhance our running more than any of our current alternative sports." His hunch is probably on the money. The question is, How do we penetrate the closed minds of the runners and get them to try an innovative training mix of walking and running?

According to Dr. Sheehan, Coach Andrews, whose athletes included cyclists, never advised his runners to cycle as part of their training. In fact, his world record holder Shrubb warned runners against cycling, saying that it tends to "chop" the stride. Whether cycling "chops" the stride or not, it is a proven fact that world-class cyclists or swimmers cannot transfer their aerobic capacity to running the way the U.S. and Mexican race walkers did.

In the last chapter, I cited a study in which trained swimmers who were tested on a treadmill running test showed *no* aerobic improvement when running. If there is no aerobic cross-training effect between swimming and running, then why is swimming recommended as a cross-training exercise for runners and high-intensity walking not?

I suspect the reason is a combination of two things: the blind contempt that runners have for the walking gait and the lack of physiological testing of the walking gait by runners at speeds beyond the 12-minute-mile metabolic intersection. Unfortunately, that testing can't happen unless runners change their attitudes, as we found out at the USOTC.

Dr. Sheehan had no idea what was under way at the USOTC when he wrote the closing sentence of his column: "I hope our exercise physiologists will take it upon themselves to demonstrate scientifically what the great Harry Andrews found in practice: Walking and running are no more than two forms of the same activity." His hope has been fulfilled. Now the new knowledge needs to be applied to various training regimens.

The study by Drs. Byrnes and Kearney demonstrated scientifically that high-intensity walkers not only achieved maximum oxygen uptakes similar to those of runners but also could *switch to running and achieve the same oxygen uptakes without cross-training*. What is the significance of this apparent aberration in the specificity principle? It is obvious that high-intensity walking should play a major role in a wide variety of sports and athletic aerobic-conditioning regimens. Indeed, where walking has previously been universally excluded from intense aerobic training, we may find that more walking and less running will produce better athletes *with fewer injuries*.

I am convinced that there are unlimited physical-conditioning possibilities with high-intensity aerobic walking. Let's contemplate a few hypothetical training regimens for a variety of athletic circumstances.

DO RUNNERS NEED AEROBIC WALKING?

In the days of Harry Andrews and Alfie Shrubb, aerobic conditioning, interval training, and cross-training were unknown. Highly sophisticated equipment to test athletic fitness didn't exist. Much of what was done by coaches and athletes was done by feel and instinct. By today's standards, it was the Stone Age of exercise physiology.

Nevertheless, those early coaches and athletes must have instinctively understood that their approach helped reduce injuries, the bane of all runners. I believe reintroducing walking—specifically high-intensity aerobic walking—into runners' training schedules may produce two major benefits: the opportunity to (1) reduce injuries; (2) maintain a high aerobic capacity by converting a large share of "junk miles" (which simply burn calories and keep body fat down) to aerobic walking miles in order to take advantage of walking's unique capacity to transfer aerobic fitness to running. The ultimate reduction of impact on the musculoskeletal system would be impressive.

A look at some conservative theoretical numbers will reveal how impressive. In *Exercise Physiology*, for convenient comparisons and evaluations of body build and composition, a "reference man and reference woman" is developed by Albert Behnke. These are theoretical models based on average physical dimensions. The reference man is 20 to 24 years old and weighs 154 pounds. The reference woman is in the same age range and weighs 125 pounds.

For a theoretical runner's training schedule, let's assume that the reference man currently runs 40 miles a week, including interval training. If half of this was converted to high-intensity aerobic walking, what would be the reduction of impact to his musculoskeletal system in one week with *no sacrifice to aerobic conditioning*?

The average runner hits the ground at 3.50 times his or her body weight. A walker loads his weight onto his foot at 1.25 to 1.50 times his body weight. Any analysis of the two gaits must take into account the way the foot makes contact with the ground. A runner is airborne, and his heel strikes the ground, introducing shock to the musculoskeletal system. By contrast, a walker is always in contact with the ground, and his heel is placed on it without impact. That is significant. A runner on each step will hit the ground with a force at least 2 times his body weight more than a walker's (3.50 − 1.50 = 2).

Since we are using hypothetical numbers, let's assume that our reference man has a 4-foot running stride, which means he would take 1,320 steps per mile (5,280 feet ÷ 4 = 1,320). Because of the horizontal springing action of running, as a rule runners take fewer strides per mile than walkers. Pulling all the numbers together looks like this:

2 × 154 pounds = 308 extra running-impact pounds per step over walking
308 × 1,320 steps = 406,560 extra running-impact pounds per mile over walking
406,560 × 20 miles = 8,131,200 extra running-impact pounds per week over walking

Simply stated, by converting half of his running time to aerobic walking, the runner in the example would have reduced the trauma he puts onto his musculoskeletal system by 8,131,200 pounds in just one week!

It stands to reason that over the many years of a runner's racing career (usually starting in high school), reduction of impact of this magnitude would be a significant mitigating factor in injury prevention. Indeed, high-intensity aerobic walking could not only contribute to injury prevention in runners but could very well extend some running careers. It is probably the most overlooked, underrated training option available to runners. Creative coaches should get their runners out of the swimming pools, off the cycles, and out on the road or track doing high-intensity walking for the best cross-training exercise.

Alfie Shrubb may have been more observant than modern-day coaches when he said that cycling "chops" the stride of runners. Watch the action of the leg muscles, particularly the hamstrings, on a cyclist. They never get fully extended in a full rotation of the pedals. The hamstrings were biomechanically engineered over millions of years of evolution to function for walking and running, not cycling. Getting those muscles ready for running by cycling is counter to the specificity principle. It would be interesting to know whether runners who cycle a lot suffer more pulled hamstrings than those who don't. It is something to think about.

Something else to think about is why run-cycle biathlons are being promoted instead of walk-run biathlons? Now that we know that high-intensity walking complements the aerobic capacity of a runner, doesn't it follow that if runners start to train with walking, some of them will get very good at it? Isn't the most obvious biathlon of all a walk-run, in which the athlete must excel in his or her *two natural gaits*?

COULD JACK NICKLAUS WIN THE MASTERS AGAIN?

From a pure application of the specificity principle, perhaps no group of athletes could get more out of high-intensity aerobic walking than the professional golfers on the PGA and LPGA tours. It would do for them what no other exercise can. Until I started researching this book, I had no idea that these highly paid professional athletes are still in the Dark Ages when it comes to proper conditioning for one of the most grueling physical and mental challenges in all of professional sports.

Why does an Arnold Palmer, a Jack Nicklaus, or a Tom Watson suddenly stop winning big tournaments and some young shooters fresh out of nowhere start knocking them off? Practically all professional golfers rely solely on their natural talent, backed up with dedicated attention to hand-eye coordination. They relentlessly practice driving, chipping, and putting, but spend no time on conditioning their walking gait, which must carry them through a long tournament. Young legs will beat tired old legs every time, in just about every sport.

The PGA and LPGA have highly equipped, well-staffed fitness-training vehicles that follow their tours. On May 8, 1991, I spoke with Rob Mottram, an exercise physiologist who had worked the fitness vehicle for the LPGA tour for three years but was now working the PGA tour. He told me that there were about 150 male golfers on the tour, and that each round of golf requires the golfer to be on his feet for four or five hours constantly, without ever sitting down. The same is true for the women.

Mottram explained that a typical four-day tournament is usually preceded by a one-day pro-am round, which often lasts longer than five hours. What kind of conditioning do the golfers practice

for this grueling schedule? Practically *none* that would contribute
to their walking gait, which has to carry them through the tournament. According to Mottram, about 15 percent of the male
golfers do some jogging; 3 miles several days a week was typical.
On a sporadic basis, 10 percent use an exercise cycle and about 25
percent use a climbing device for cardiovascular conditioning. Mottram said that about two thirds of them do some stretching and
flexibility exercises.

With such a lack of proper physical conditioning of the walking
gait, it is not surprising to see Jack Nicklaus, in my view the greatest
golfer of all time, admit to *USA Today*: "I just ran out of gas"
when he shot a 76 on the last round of the 1991 Masters. Earlier
in the tournament, on fresher legs, he had a sizzling 66. With his
superior talent and a high-intensity walking program, I believe
Nicklaus should be able to win many more big tournaments. But
he has to *start* with a full tank of gas. On TV, when I watched
him trudge up to the eighteenth hole on the last day of the Masters,
I could tell by his stride that he was leg weary.

Pro golfers take the walking gait for granted. A younger Palmer,
Nicklaus, or Watson only had to concentrate on perfecting his
game; walking on young legs made it easy. Now as for an aging
boxer, baseball player, or basketball player, the legs become a
factor in performance for these tournament golfers. It becomes
more difficult to hold the fragile parameters of a perfect golf swing
together with aging, unconditioned, fatigued torso-support and
leg-propulsion muscles. These muscles reveal their lack of conditioning when drives find the rough, sand traps seem to be in the
wrong place, and putts break left instead of right.

For a tournament golfer, the subtleties of fatigue in the walking
gait are deceptive. Everything else is questioned when the game
unravels. Just because the golfer is upright and able to trudge along,
no one suspects that those unconditioned major muscle groups
responsible for posture, balance, and propulsion, which are an
integral part of every successful golf swing, could be responsible.
Remedies for a bad round are sought on the driving range and on
the putting green instead of on the road.

Older players like Nicklaus and Watson who still show flashes
of their former brilliance are prime candidates for high-intensity
aerobic walking. Younger players who find their game falling apart
on the third or fourth day of a tournament may also soon find
that a well-conditioned walking gait would add coordinated con-

sistency to their game. A high-intensity walking regimen of 3 to 5 miles at least four days a week would give Nicklaus a pair of legs that would carry him through a tournament without fatigue.

In addition, a pro golfer would find that high-intensity walking has a residual benefit that running, exercise cycles, or climbing devices don't provide. High-intensity aerobic walking makes the exerciser focus his or her mind over the entire distance of the walk. The walker has to coordinate all the major muscle groups from the neck down into one fluid, coordinated athletic move, which is exactly what a golfer does on a golf swing. It requires total concentration to hold the fast pace. It not only produces physical toughness but heightened mental concentration.

The effectiveness of high-intensity walking for women golfers might be even greater. Women are such natural walkers that not only would such training work for them but they would enjoy it. Every woman I know who has taken up aerobic walking says that it elevates her energy level, mental acuity, and personal confidence. There is reason to believe that players in both the PGA and the LPGA could possibly win tournaments more consistently if they got physically fit and mentally tough for grueling tournament play with high-intensity aerobic walking.

GETTING READY TO GO 15 ROUNDS

Dr. Sheehan listed boxers among the athletes who trained by the Andrews walking method at the turn of the century. I'd like to introduce a few boxers to "Casey's Walking Method." Boxers must condition the lower *and* upper body to withstand fatigue over 10, 12, or 15 rounds of concentrated physical exertion. Often, however, they aren't conditioned to go the distance, and in the late rounds weary arms and legs take their toll. Mike Tyson is a perfect example of a superior fighter losing to a lesser rival for all the wrong reasons.

From what I have read, a boxer's road work consists primarily of jogging for aerobic conditioning. In the *Rocky* series, Sylvester Stallone dramatized the running aspects of his training. But a boxer could get upper- *and* lower-body fitness in about 50 minutes a day with high-intensity walking. The concentrated rhythmic physical activity of all the major muscle groups from the neck down would give him the stamina he needs to go 15 rounds at full power.

Done in conjunction with his other training, a hypothetical

eight-week, high-intensity aerobic-walking training regimen for a boxer might go like this:

Walk five days a week, 5 miles each day, at a 10-minute-mile pace. Total: 50 minutes per day. At an estimated 3-foot stride that would be 1,760 steps and 1,760 arm swings per mile (5,280 feet ÷ 3 = 1,760).

ARM SWINGS. The aerobic walker's bent-arm swing is short and powerful, much like that of a boxer throwing a body punch. At 1,760 steps per mile, the boxer would swing his arms 8,800 times per 5-mile workout (1,760 × 5 = 8,800). In eight weeks (40 days) of high-intensity walking, the boxer would have performed 352,000 short, powerful arm swings (8,800 × 40 = 352,000). Weights in half-pound increments would be added the last four weeks, as long as the boxer could maintain his walking speed with controlled posture, rhythm, and technique. (I am adamantly opposed to hand weights except for this type of training, for reasons given in Chapter 11.)

LEG CONDITIONING. While the arms are counterbalancing the legs with 352,000 pistonlike swings, all the major muscle groups in the lower body are firing to propel the boxer along with an equal number of leg swings. The chance of a boxer becoming leg weary in 15 rounds after a training regimen of high-intensity walking is rather remote.

CONCENTRATION. This level of aerobic walking would force the boxer to focus his mind for 50 minutes—and that's 5 minutes longer than a 15-round fight. Such training would enhance his concentration.

FOOTBALL PLAYERS: TOO BIG TO JOG

In 1986, when I was writing my first book, William "The Refrigerator" Perry, the big lineman for the Chicago Bears, had just burst on the scene. He was something of an oddity at the time because of his impressive size, which was over 300 pounds. Today it seems that most NFL linemen are routinely stamped out by a 300-pound cookie cutter. Even NCAA Division 1 linemen at that weight are not unusual. I can think of few athletes who could use high-intensity aerobic walking better. Most of them have had invasive knee surgery even before leaving college. The standard use of jogging to develop aerobic conditioning puts unnecessary trauma onto their musculoskeletal systems, and it probably shortens their highly paid careers.

In an earlier section of this chapter, I used Dr. Albert Behnke's reference man as a basis for age and weight in my example of how much concussion a runner puts onto his musculoskeletal system when running. In this example I will use "Casey's Reference NFL Lineman." Let's assume he is 23 to 26 years old, weighs an even 300 pounds, and is going to jog for 28 days before going to football camp for basic aerobic fitness.

A review of the pounds of impact he will put on his musculo-skeletal system staggers the mind. Remember that a runner hits the ground with a force that is 3.5 times his body weight. Here are the numbers:

300 pounds × 3.5 = 1,050 impact pounds per step
1,320 steps × 1,050 = 1,386,000 impact pounds per mile
3 miles × 1,386,000 = 4,158,000 impact pounds per day
28 days × 4,158,000 = 116,424,000 impact pounds total

This last number is the impact the lineman has subjected his musculoskeletal system to—and he hasn't even put his football pads on yet. The bigger and heavier the athlete, the more important it is to reduce the long-term cumulative effect of jogging's impact on the musculoskeletal system. There has to be a better way, and the aerobic conditioning of high-intensity walking is it.

While I have used linemen in this example, franchise players, such as quarterbacks Joe Montana and Dan Marino, need aerobic walking even more. Montana has had a serious back injury that required surgery. Bad backs don't take kindly to jogging. Marino has had knee surgery and plays with a knee brace. These multi-million-dollar players are vital to their team's success. They must have a high degree of physical fitness to survive the pounding and fatigue that constitutes their normal working day, and no other exercise or exercise equipment can give them a better injury-free physical fitness than high-intensity aerobic walking.

NAVRATILOVA, JORDAN, AND OTHERS

Martina Navratilova, world champion tennis player, is in the twilight of her career. Superstar Michael Jordan, the heart and soul of the 1990 NBA Champion Chicago Bulls, is at the height of his. One thing they have in common, however, even though they are in quite different sports and at different stages of their careers, is deteriorating knees. Over the past few years, Navratilova's knees have finally succumbed to the abrupt stopping, starting, and twisting lateral moves that are part of tennis. At the beginning of the 1991 NBA season, it was reported that Jordan was starting to experience knee problems. As of this writing those problems do not appear to be serious, but in time many professional basketball players eventually yield to career-ending leg and foot injuries. That's simply part of the turf in the NBA. The injury-healing process does not respond as well as athletes age, and performance ultimately suffers.

Whether it's Navratilova, Jordan, Montana, or Marino, athletes who are of championship caliber know they must go into each game in the best physical condition possible to perform at a peak level. In addition, a high level of physical fitness forestalls fatigue, which is the precursor to even more injuries. Battling an aging body and trying to stay fit without putting more trauma onto a musculoskeletal system that cannot stand any more is the dilemma facing the Navratilovas and Jordans of professional sports. These are two classic instances in which high-intensity walking could help squeeze a few more years out of some battered knees and extend the careers of these popular athletes who are already legends in their games.

FROM THE ATHLETIC FIELD TO THE BATTLEFIELD

In the winter of 1991, I was glued to the TV with the rest of the nation watching Operation Desert Storm. It renewed my interest in the physical condition of our ground troops. My interest was heightened because of a letter I had received in July 1989 from a lieutenant colonel who was director of training for the infantry. I do not wish to embarrass him, so I will not use his name.

I had contacted him by telephone after I read in *USA Today* that the army was trying to train its recruits by using aerobics classes to reduce injuries from running. He seemed somewhat flustered by the story and indicated that it was merely experimental. Not long after my call, however, *The Wall Street Journal* ran a story under the heading "And the Mess Hall's Lunch Menu Offers

Spinach Quiche and Yogurt." It was a tongue-in-cheek poke at the army and the marines.

The story read: "Say It Ain't So—Yes, It's True: Aerobics Is Now Part of the Military's Physical Regimen." There were differing opinions about the effectiveness of aerobics in the military. Staff Sargeant William E. Grant, an outspoken infantryman, said, "Aerobics are for wimps, plain and simple. . . . This kind of activity does not build strong soldiers mentally and physically." First Lieutenant Arnold Kozoloski, a Marine Corps public-relations officer, told the paper: "So many soldiers were getting hurt, the military developed an exercise program that works muscles smarter, not necessarily harder."

I had written the lieutenant colonel a lengthy letter explaining gait efficiency and the specificity-of-training advantage that high-intensity walking has over running for the physical conditioning of an infantry soldier. I even offered to put on a clinic for him. In his reply he said that the army encourages walking, but "it is used mainly for profiled overweight and more senior soldiers." After that cold shower, it was all downhill, with comments like "Running is more performance oriented" and "Cardiovascular benefits for normal populations are realized sooner using a running program." The comment that really got me riled was "Running is a more natural exercise." More natural than walking?

There are few instances in which a high-intensity walking program could make a better direct contribution to a specifically needed level of physical fitness than that of an infantry soldier. Forced marches and battlefield conditions require fit legs and a properly conditioned walking gait. The running gait and aerobic routines contribute little or nothing to cross-training for walking.

Another reason that high-intensity walking makes sense for the military is the number of women in the services. CNN reported that there were 35,000 women in Operation Desert Storm. I find that women almost universally dislike running, but that they are sensational walkers.

With high-intensity walking, it would be much simpler to turn out a highly fit soldier, male or female, with fewer injuries. For instance, a combination of about 70 percent high-intensity aerobic walking and 30 percent running should significantly reduce injuries. It would produce a soldier who could not only run to the army's current standards but also walk at a level that the army and marines don't even yet comprehend. From a functional standpoint, at war or peace, the latter is more important. Any young recruit who can't do what I call the *triple nickel* (walk 5 miles in 55 minutes) shouldn't graduate from basic training. Furthermore, any senior combat officer who can't do the *triple triple* (walk 3 miles in 33 minutes) should be put out to pasture. At 64 years of age, I am still able to do both.

THE MOST IMPORTANT CHAPTER IN THIS BOOK

While I was writing this book a friend asked, "What could conceivably be new and exciting about walking?" Without hesitation I said, "Read Chapter 8. It's the most important one in the book and could possibly revolutionize athletic training." I believe that the study at the USOTC is more impressive for what it left unanswered than for what it demonstrated. When Bill Byrnes was explaining the data in Vancouver, he said, "This study may only be the tip of the iceberg for high-intensity walking as an athletic training aid. . . . What we need now are more scientific studies to track performance results and hopefully injury reduction and experimentation by coaches and athletes in various sports using high-intensity walking as part of their training regimen."

The last words in the NaturalSport cross-training study abstract—"indicates a potential cross-training effect"—could have an explosive impact on athletic conditioning. Even though Drs. Byrnes and Kearney worded this premise cautiously, one only has to look at Figure 8.2 to see that the oxygen uptake was higher in every instance in the running gait for walkers. Although the higher figure is not large enough to be statistically significant, the fact that they could duplicate it in both gaits without cross-training is truly remarkable.

The NaturalSport cross-training study demonstrated that high-intensity walking *can transfer all its oxygen uptake level to running, and no other exercise can do that.* It is clearly an aberration in the specificity principle that cries out for experimentation and implementation by exercise physiologists, coaches, and athletes. It opens up a wide range of new training possibilities that could lead to better athletic performance, extended athletic careers, reduction of training-induced injuries, and faster recovery of aerobic fitness for running after an injury.

Using hypothetical training regimens, I have boldly suggested how runners, professional golfers, boxers, football players, and others, including the infantry and marines, could benefit from high-intensity aerobic walking. In addition, Dr. George Sheehan's highly respected voice has urged further study of walking as a training aid. It is time to try this revolutionary approach to athletic conditioning. It would be a shame if experimentation and implementation were held back by the intellectuals and scholars—i.e., coaches, athletes, and colonels—who still believe that the sun revolves around the earth.

9

RACE WALKING: THE ULTIMATE ATHLETIC CHALLENGE

The Friday, May 31, 1991, issue of *USA Today* typified the sorry state of race walking in this country. In San Jose, California, over 300 race walkers from more than 30 countries were in town for the weekend to compete in the Race Walking World Cup races (20K and 50K for men; 10K for women), which are held in different countries every two years. In terms of international significance, these races are second only to the Olympic Games.

Most of the international race-walking champions and active world record holders were in San Jose. Many will compete in the 1992 summer Olympics at Barcelona, Spain. They are the cream of the crop. *USA Today* prides itself on covering important events in the nation and spotting trends, but its Friday sports section, which listed major sporting events for that weekend, did not give the Race Walking World Cup a single line of type.

The ultimate irony of this omission occurred in the same issue of *USA Today*, even more ironically, in their sports section. The paper reported that the latest tabulations on exercise popularity showed that "the USA's No. 1 recreational sport is walking. Total walkers: 71.4 million, up 72% since 1985." That number is more than three times the number of runners and joggers in this country and is growing every year.

Except for the *San Jose Mercury News*, no major paper gave the World Cup any prerace coverage. A TV crew from Japan was there. The Japanese have a good 50K race walker, but most of their other walkers are not serious international contenders. The men's 20K and women's 10K races were on Saturday, June 1, but ABC's *Wide World of Sport* chose instead to cover a mini-marathon, which is not even a regulation track and field event.

I believe that race walking is either ignored or subjected to ridicule as a sport for the same reason that walking has been ignored as an exercise. Since walkers don't go as fast as runners, walking has not been taken seriously as an exercise or as a sport. Exercise physiologists and sports reporters seem to focus on speed and don't realize that walking and running are distinct gaits, with totally different biomechanical characteristics and degrees of difficulty.

The ridicule directed at race walking obviously comes from the technique the walkers use to achieve their phenomenal speeds. Most sportswriters and commentators who make lame attempts at humor about the technique don't have the foggiest idea how the biomechanics of the walking gait works. They don't really know how the running gait works either, but they assume that since it is faster it must be a greater athletic challenge. That is not a very cerebral approach, which indicates that their coverage is as shallow as their knowledge. What is it about race walking that makes it the least understood of all the track and field events? Let's take a look.

RACE WALKING EXPLAINED

Chapter 5 covered the correct posture for *all* walkers—strollers, brisk, aerobic, and race. Chapter 6 introduced aerobic walking and the bent-arm swing so you could increase your arm swing to match your increased stride frequency as you pick up the pace of your walk. At this point you are already two thirds of the way to becoming a race walker. Learning the lower-body movements is the other third and the cause of much comment.

First, let me disqualify myself as a race-walking expert. I am an avid race-walking fan, however, and, through my research and contacts, I have access to the experts. For this chapter, I have the advice and counsel of a longtime friend, Leonard Jansen, who helped me with my first book. Jansen was head of computer services at the Sports Science Division of the USOTC. As an analyst at their biomechanics lab, he has viewed and analyzed miles of film and videotape of the internationally ranked race walkers, including the world-record-setting Russians and Mexicans. Jansen is the foremost authority in the United States on the current state of the art of world-class race walking.

Essentially, what race walkers do with the lower body is to flex the pelvis forward as their non-weight-bearing legs swing out in front of them toward heel plant. As the pelvis reaches maximum forward flexion, it tilts down, lowering the body's center of mass as the heel is placed on the ground. This simple biomechanical maneuver accomplishes two things: (1) it lengthens the walker's stride; (2) it lowers the body's center of mass to reduce the rising and falling of the body on each step, so the walker can achieve more efficient forward progression.

As Dr. Inman explains in his analysis of the human walking gait, which was cited in Chapter 5, each walker has some natural pelvic rotation on the non-weight-bearing side of the forward swinging leg. He also points out that this rotation increases with walking speed. Race walkers intentionally increase their forward pelvic flexion to bring the hip joint of the swinging leg farther forward, contributing to greater stride length.

As the pelvis is being flexed forward, it is also developing what Dr. Inman calls a "pelvic list." It is tilted down away from the weight-bearing leg; thus the body's hypothetical center of mass (located in the pelvis) is lowered. In his analysis of this phase of the walking gait, Dr. Inman states: "As the walking speed increases, there is a progressive increase in the amount of drop of the pelvis to the side of the leg in the swing phase." He adds, "At higher speeds, the pelvis is not lifted all the way to a level position during the latter part of the swing phase." Race walkers use this unique biomechanical feature of the walking gait to reduce the normal vertical rising and falling of the body, which are counterproductive for forward progression.

The forward flexion of the pelvis and the subsequent downward pelvic list create an unusual visual effect that is not associated with regular walking. Sadly, this necessary biomechanical action causes sportswriters and commentators to make inane remarks about it. They often stereotype it as a side-to-side wiggle, which it is not. The description I have given you may sound relatively simple, but putting it into practice along with the other subtleties and nuances of the race-walking technique requires years of training before a walker can reach top competitive speeds.

To get a quick idea of how the pelvis flexes forward and lists at the same time, stand with both feet under you, knees fully flexed and locked. Keeping one leg flexed and locked, snap the other knee forward and watch your hip on that side quickly flex forward and tilt down. While you are standing with both feet on the ground, rotate your pelvis forward and backward a few times. As your pelvis flexes forward, you can observe about how much it would contribute to your stride length if you were doing this movement in conjunction with your leg swing.

Now that you understand the biomechanics of how the walking stride can be efficiently lengthened, take a few extralong steps the conventional way, simply swinging your legs farther out in front, as recommended in some other walking books. You will quickly notice that there is an unrhythmic rising and falling of your body. Lengthening the stride this way would not make for an enjoyable walk and would certainly not allow you to increase your speed. The only way to lengthen stride and increase speed in a fluid, rhythmic manner is the way race walkers do it.

The forward flexion of the pelvis also enables the race walker to achieve in-line foot placement. This virtually eliminates lateral sway of the upper body, which affects speed. It also lessens strain on the groin muscles at racing speeds. Normal walking leaves two parallel tracks, as shown in Figure 9.1A. As you learned in Chapter 5, people who track wide when they walk have noticeable lateral upper-body sway. Race walkers eliminate this by walking with a single track, shown in Figure 9.1B.

To give you a better idea of the pelvis's role in this biomechanical maneuver, Figure 9.2A shows a cutaway top view of the pelvis in a normal walking stride. The feet land in parallel tracks, and the pelvis is squared to the line of travel. Figure 9.2B shows the forward flexion of a race walker's pelvis on the right side with the feet landing on line. If this illustration could be done in three dimensions, it would also reveal that the right hip is lower than the left. With the trailing foot almost directly behind the center of mass (see black square), and with the center of mass also lower, race walkers can maximize forward thrust and minimize vertical oscillation of the body. Thus they are able to walk with exceptional speed.

FIGURE 9.1A

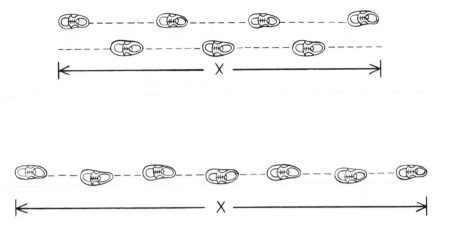

FIGURE 9.1B

Jansen, who also coached our World Cup team, points out that today's walkers' faster times probably result from a changed emphasis on stride length. He explains that in years past the walker reached as far forward as possible with the swing leg. At heel plant, when the body is momentarily in the double-stance phase, the legs formed a near-isosceles triangle (having two equal sides), as shown in Figure 9.3A. Note that the lines from the center of mass down the legs to the front foot and back foot are roughly equal. Each foot is also equidistant from the vertical line of gravity at the center of mass.

Figure 9.3B shows the new style, in which the front foot is placed closer to the line of gravity at the center of mass and the trailing foot is farther from it. This position permits the heel to be planted quickly and smoothly. More important, it reduces the time that the leg is in front of the center of mass (when it is a resistance to forward progression) and increases the time that the foot is behind the walker pushing against the ground for forward thrust. I think you will agree that the complex biomechanics of the race-walking technique are far more involved than meets the untrained eye.

The way race walkers plant their heels and load their weight onto their feet is also important. When the swing leg reaches its maximum forward extension, it is straight at the knee. The toes

FIGURE 9.2A   **FIGURE 9.2B**

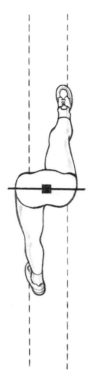
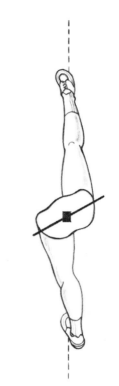

are up at a comfortable angle. When the heel is placed on the ground, the foot should be in a supinated position (turned outward or laterally). As it is lowered to the ground, the foot rolls forward along the outside edge to the ball of the foot and then to toe-off (see Figure 9.4). The leg should remain straight at the knee from heel plant through the weight-bearing phase to toe-off.

Chapter 6 recommended that aerobic walkers place their feet on the ground with a slight emphasis on the outside edge. Race walkers, by contrast, come down on the outside edges of their feet in a pronounced manner when they load their weight. To do this properly requires coaching and a lot of practice. I recommend that you do not attempt to walk with an abnormally supinated foot placement without coaching. You will not like it, you won't be able to walk any faster, and you might injure yourself.

A race walker leans slightly forward from the ankles; the back

FIGURE 9.3A

FIGURE 9.3B

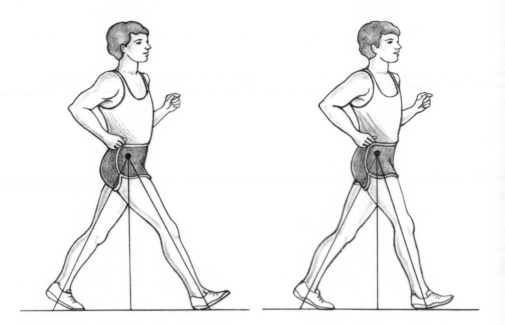

FIGURE 9.4

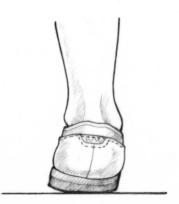

is straight from the ankles to the ears, never bent at the waist. Utilizing the bent-arm swing in combination with pelvic flexion and listing, the walker develops a smooth, rhythmic, coordinated move. The pelvis should flex back and forth on each step with no side-to-side wiggle.

As each leg swings forward under the body, it should be bent at the knee just enough for the foot to clear the ground. The heel of the front foot should land directly in line with the toe of the back foot. A properly coached and trained race walker literally skims across the ground, with every biomechanical move of the arms, hips, legs, and feet carefully coordinated to produce a highly efficient rhythmic, fluid, forward progression. All the major muscle groups in the legs and pelvic area are used to power the walker along at phenomenal speeds. Race walking requires the flexibility of a gymnast, the grace of a dancer, and the endurance of a marathon runner. I will state flatly that I believe it requires more mental and physical discipline and far more coordinated athletic ability to become a world-class race walker than to become a world-class runner.

It should now be apparent why I separate race walking from exercise walking. To be a serious contender in a competitive field takes considerable coaching and training to master the race-walking technique. Merely walking a little faster than normal with bent arms is hardly race walking. Good race walkers walk faster than a 10-minute-mile pace. However, if you are an older person, you can win many races in the 10- to 12-minute-mile range. Aerobic walking will take you to this level, and you won't have to learn the complex lower-body movements of race walking. I walk in this range at the ripe old age of 64.

RACE-WALKING RULES

Whether you master the race-walking technique or simply use the bent-arm-swing aerobic-walking technique to compete, two rules must be observed. The first is the double-contact rule, which requires the heel of the front foot to touch the ground before the toe of the back foot leaves the ground (see the brackets in Figure 9.5). This is simple enough to understand because, as you learned in Chapter 3, any time you have both feet off the ground at the same time you are running.

The other rule requires that when the weight-bearing leg passes

FIGURE 9.5

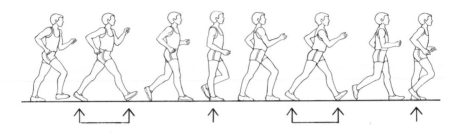

under the body it must be momentarily fully straightened at the knee. The single arrow in Figure 9.5 points to the race walker's straightened weight-bearing leg. The straight knee is somewhat difficult for ex-runners to master because they are used to running with bent knees. I use the straight knee on my daily walks because I find it gives me a rhythmic, rolling gait. It is something you should practice as an aerobic walker, even if you don't compete. Do not snap the knee back and hyperextend it; simply bring it to a fully straightened position.

In a judged race, a walker can be disqualified (DQ) if he or she receives three DQ cards from three different judges. Four to eight judges are used in a race, with one head judge chosen from the group. A "runner" (usually on a bicycle or motorbike) circulates among the judges and picks up DQ cards. Each judge has a paddle with the symbol for the bent leg (creeping) on one side and for loss of contact (lifting) on the other (see Figure 9.6). A judge may—but isn't required to—issue a warning to a walker by flashing the appropriate symbol at the athlete before he or she finally issues a DQ card. If a walker receives three DQ cards during the race, the head judge finds the athlete on the course as soon as possible. He or she holds a red flag in front of the walker to disqualify the contestant and says something like "Number 78, Jack Jones, you have been disqualified. Please remove your number and leave the course." Judging is an important part of race walking, and there is a national shortage of judges.

Figure 9.7A shows a race walker in a series of steps with the knees bent (see arrows). Figure 9.7B shows a race walker with a loss-of-contact violation (see brackets). The sport can't grow as fast as it should at all levels until more judges are available. It is

FIGURE 9.6A

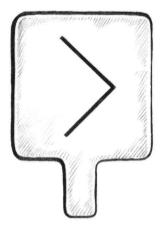

FIGURE 9.6B

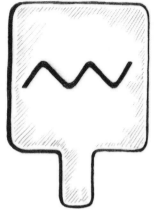

FIGURE 9.7A

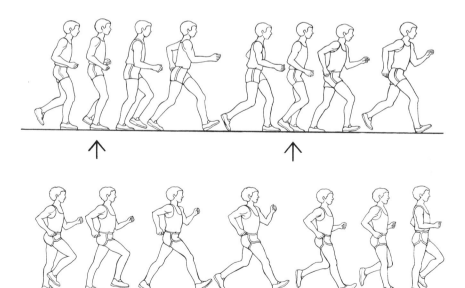

FIGURE 9.7B

not difficult to pass the test to become certified. Actually, the hardest part is gaining experience so that you can spot someone who is lifting or creeping. If you would like to become a certified race-walking judge (you do not have to be a race walker), contact Elaine Ward, managing director of the nonprofit North American Race Walking Foundation, P.O. Box 50312, Pasadena, CA 91115-0312, phone (818) 577-2264. Ward will send you the information you need to get started. Other challenging athletic contests that are judged events are gymnastics, diving, and figure skating. They require great skill and athletic coordination, just like race walking.

Race walking needs more people, young, middle-aged, and old, to take up the sport. Unfortunately, there is no feeder system for race walking. It is not a high school track and field event; consequently, it is not an NCAA university and college sport. Because it is poorly understood and often unfairly maligned by sportswriters, many people who would like to give it a try refrain from fear of ridicule. I am sure this will soon change. A lot of those 71 million exercise walkers out there are going to want to find out how fast they can walk, just as some joggers wanted to find out how fast they could run.

RACE WALKING'S HIGH DEGREE OF DIFFICULTY

If a track and field meet is examined on a degree-of-difficulty basis, race walking should be one of the premier events. Race walking is as difficult as any other track event, and its required athletic coordination exceeds most of the others.

Track and field events are made up of many arbitrarily devised physical challenges that have no relevance to the scheme of life—for example, the triple jump, pole vault, shotput, discus, javelin, high jump, hammer throw, and hurdles. What is so intriguing about seeing how far someone can pitch a heavy ball or throw a discus? There are critics who say race walking doesn't make sense because running is faster. If that's the case, why have hurdles? Why not go around them; wouldn't that be faster?

Degree of athletic difficulty is an important element in every sports event. Anyone who has watched Greg Louganis do his complicated, twisting gold-medal-winning dives in the Olympics would have to agree. Using the analogy that running is better because it gets you from Point A to Point B faster, Louganis could save himself a lot of time and training if he just held his nose and dove straight into the water. Isn't it strange how degree of difficulty is applauded in one judged sporting event and ridiculed in another?

Way back in the preface, I said that walking and running must be understood as gaits before they can be understood as exercise and sport. There are two gaits of horse racing, and they have a parallel in humans. Trotting horses pull a sulky and take the trotting gait to phenomenal speeds. The world record for the mile is 1:52 1/5. Humans don't have a trotting gait; when we became bipeds, we lost that. A race walker does essentially what a trotting horse does, however, when he or she extends the walking gait well into the speed range of a runner while resisting the compelling temptation to break stride and run. This is one of the aspects of race walking that make it such a challenging sport. It is the same ability that we admire in a good trotting horse.

I am convinced that race walking will explode in the nineties. It is the sport associated with the nation's and the world's most popular exercise, and it is the next logical step. I believe there is already a change in the wind, and, while the press and TV are still mesmerized with running, millions of walkers are starting to get curious about the sport associated with their exercise.

On Saturday morning at the World Cup races in San Jose, *Prevention* magazine mistakenly scheduled my lecture and clinic at 9:00 A.M., the time the men's 20K race was to start. The *Prevention* walkers' rally had drawn 5,000 exercise walkers from all over the United States and four foreign countries. Most of these people had never seen a race walk and, as I headed into the auditorium, which was opposite the starting line, three women averaging about age 60 asked if I would delay the lecture 15 minutes so they could watch the start of the race. Others coming in made the same request, so I put up a Postponed sign and we all watched the start. At 9:15 A.M., I had 300 people at my lecture, most of them in their fifties. When I asked for a show of hands, more than half indicated that they had never seen a walking race before. All of them thought it was exciting. I cut my lecture down to 45 minutes so we could see the last part of the race, which was won by the Russian champion Mikhail Schennikov in 1 hour, 20 minutes, and 43 seconds. Sadly, no American finished in the top 50.

REIGNING CHAMPIONS AND OLYMPIC HOPEFULS

The first race walk I ever attended was in 1985 in Denver. Two women who competed that day stand out in my mind because they both finished near last but today are reigning champions. The first was Debbie Lawrence from Kansas City, Missouri, only 50 miles from where I live. Carol and I rooted for her, but Lawrence, who was 24 years old and struggling to learn the race-walking technique, finished poorly. Today, with dedication and disciplined training, she holds the American 10K track record in 46:10.26 and the 10K road record in 45:34. She was named Woman Walker of the Year in 1990.

The other walker was a 6-foot-tall woman in her midthirties named Viisha Sedlak. Being tall is not necessarily an asset in race walking, and in those days Sedlak had a gawky, stork-like walk. You should see her now; in her early forties, Sedlak is a smooth, fluid, well-oiled walking machine. At the 1990 *Prevention* spring walkers' rally in Tampa, Florida, Sedlak not only won the open 5K citizens' race but beat two nationally ranked Masters male walkers. She holds double World Masters records (over 40), the 5K in 24:38, and the 10K road record in 49:14.9. Sedlak is now ranked the World's Number 1 Masters Women walker.

The story of Debbie Lawrence and Viisha Sedlak is indicative of the time it takes to truly master the race-walking technique. Years of practice and training are required to go from walking at the back of the pack to becoming a record-breaking champion. People who think race walking at the speeds these walkers achieve is not an enormous athletic accomplishment haven't tried it.

In 1992, the Olympic summer games will have a women's 10K race walk for the first time. Along with Debbie Lawrence, a talented walker from Sayville, New York, named Lynn Weik figures to make the three-woman team. She was Woman Walker of the Year in 1989. Weik is just 25 (Lawrence is 30) and was a close second to Lawrence when she set both of her 10K records. Weik is an extremely talented and disciplined athlete, coached by Gary Westerfield, one of the best race-walking coaches in the United States. With her combination of youth and advanced stage of development, she figures to become America's dominant female walker in the next few years.

After Lawrence and Weik, Teresa Vaill, Victoria Herazo, Michelle Rohl, Lyn Brubaker, Wendy Sharp, Debbie Van Orden, and Sara Standley are the only other contenders for the USA's first women's Olympic race-walking team. In the men's Olympic race-walking events (20K and 50K), we may not be able even to field three men for each. In the 20K, a qualifying time of 1:24 is required. As of the summer of 1991, Tim Lewis is the only American who has demonstrated the athletic ability to walk this fast. In the 50K we have just three active men walkers (Carl Schueler, Marco Evonick, and Herman Nelson) who stand a chance of meeting the qualifying time of 4:05.

For a young athlete, male or female, looking for a ticket to the Olympics, no sport offers a better opportunity than race walking. The talent pool of strong, nationally ranked race walkers is very small. Looking ahead to the 1996 Olympics, in the women's division, only Lynn Weik and Sara Standley of the current contenders will still be under 30 years of age; the rest will be in their mid-to-late thirties. In the men's division, Tim Lewis will be 33. Carl Schueler, our best 50K walker, will be 40. This sport is crying out for young athletes who want the thrill and honor of competing in the Olympics.

Mothers who have young daughters with athletic ability should direct them toward race walking. The earlier the start, the better. Race walking is virtually injury free (no shinsplints or stress fractures) and it is something they will enjoy for a lifetime. Many injured female runners become race walkers with phenomenal success. In 1987, Nadezhda Ryashkina was a struggling middle-distance Russian runner who suffered an Achilles tendon injury. She turned to race walking, and in 1990, at the Goodwill Games in Seattle, Washington, set a 10K world record in the scorching time of 41:56.21.

There is often a misconception that people with long legs will be faster walkers, but it is simply not true. Stride frequency, not stride length, determines speed. Ryashkina is only five feet, three and a half inches and weighs 101 pounds. Anna Rita Sidoti of Italy, who was ranked third in the world in 1990, is four feet, eleven and three quarters inches and weighs 88 pounds. World champion 20K walker Ernesto Canto from Mexico is only five feet, seven inches and weighs 130 pounds. His countryman Carlos Mercenario, who won the 1991 men's 50K World Cup in San Jose, is five feet, nine inches and weighs 130. Another Mexican with a big engine is Graciela Mendoza, who is all of four feet, eleven inches tall; she finished second in the 1991 women's 10K World Cup. Having a "big engine" is a lot more important for a race walker than being tall.

THE RACE WALKERS' NETWORK

Even though there are great opportunities for young athletes to win a trip to the Olympics via race walking, I'm always asked, "Where do I learn race walking, and who are the coaches?" Since race walking is not part of the school system's physical education program or track and field teams, it becomes difficult for a young walker to get proper coaching and motivation. In addition, many potential older walkers who would like to compete at a relatively modest level ask where they can get coaching and advice. The other frequent question is, "Where are the races?"

Everyone who is interested in finding out about race walking should write or call Elaine Ward at the North American Race Walking Foundation. She will send you an information packet and a list of the race-walking clubs in your area. In addition, there are a number of regional race-walking clubs that put on their own events and know where other races are taking place. Many of these clubs have good walkers who are willing to help a new race walker, (young or old) learn the technique. There isn't a friendlier, more accommodating bunch in all of sport. Get in touch with some race walkers to learn the technique; you'll make new friends and be glad you started race walking.

There are also many good newsletters on race walking and walking clubs. I can't list them all here, but I will tell you about five that I'm familiar with and recommend:

Ohio Racewalker, 3184 Summit Street, Columbus, OH 43202. This newsletter is published monthly by Jack Mortland, and it has a cultlike status among race walkers. Mortland was one of the earliest chroniclers of race walking and has published the *Ohio Racewalker* continually for 27 years. It is a 14-page booklet full of race-walking results from all over the United States, plus accounts of major races in other parts of the world. It carries news of upcoming races and discussions about various aspects of race walking. At 1991 postage rates, a yearly first-class mail subscription is only eight dollars. It's a bargain, and I look forward to it every month.

Front Range Walker's Newsletter, 2261 Glencoe Street, Denver, CO 80207. This newsletter is published by Bob Carlson, who also heads the Front Range Walkers Walking Club of Denver. The club is active in all aspects of race walking, including clinics on how to become a race-walking judge. Carlson has lots of good training information in his newsletter. I read it also.

Shore AC, 28 North Locust Street, West Long Beach, NJ 07764, c/o Elliott Denman. This is a strong East Coast club, and Denman (a 1956 Olympian), like Mortland (a 1964 Olympian), has been race walking and writing about the sport for years. He knows his stuff. Shore AC has some champion walkers, such as Ray Funkhouser, who can give you good advice on walking technique.

Pacific Pacers, 6633 NE Windemere Road, Seattle, WA 98115, c/o Bev LaVeck. My good friend Bev holds the American Women's record for the *100-mile* walk in 21 hours and 42 minutes, which she set in 1982 when she was 46. Bev is one of only four women in the United States who have walked 100 miles in less than 24 hours. Martin Rudow, former coach of the U.S. National Men's Race Walking Team, is on the board of Pacific Pacers. This is the strongest source of race-walking information and coaching in the Northwest.

Southern California Race Walking News, 1000 San Pasqual, No. 35, Pasadena, CA 91106, c/o Elaine Ward. Elaine is very active in race walking and the North American Race Walking Foundation. She will keep you informed on everything you need to know about the current state of race walking regionally and nationally.

Other active race-walking clubs are

Florida Race Walkers, c/o Henry Laskau, 3232 Carambola Circle S, Coconut Creek, FL 33066.

Georgia Race Walkers Inc., Walking Club of Georgia, c/o Dave Waddle, P.O. Box 956174, Duluth, GA 33009.

Golden State Walkers, c/o David Moore, 38623 Cherry Lane, No. 181, Fremont, CA 94536.

Heartland Race Walkers, P.O. Box 11141, Shawnee Mission, KS 66207.

Houston Race Walkers, c/o Dave Gwyn, 6502 South Briar Bayou, Houston, TX 77072.

New Mexico Walkers, c/o Gene Dix, 2301 El Nido Court, Albuquerque, NM 87104.

New Orleans Walkers, c/o New Orleans Track Club, P.O. Box 52003, New Orleans, LA 70152-2003.

Oklahoma Walkers, c/o Ron Marlett, 5736 NW 46, Oklahoma City, OK 73122.

Oregon Race Walkers, c/o Jim Bean, 4658 Fuhrer Street, NE, Salem, OR 97305.

Potomac Valley Walkers, c/o Salvatore Corrallo, 3466 Roberts Lane, North Arlington, VA 22207.

This is far from a complete list. If you are close to any of these clubs, make contact with them. Let them help you learn the race-walking technique and get involved with this growing sport. There is nothing you can do better athletically to challenge your competitive spirit in a noninjurious way and at the same time improve your ability to function in your daily life. The walking gait is so fundamental to the scheme of life for the human species that it is a mystery to me why the sports world has ignored race walking in favor of cycling, swimming, running, and contrived activities like the shot put, discus, and triple jump.

NATURALSPORT'S $50,000 RACE WALK–RUN BIATHLON

In the summer of 1991, the uncooperativeness of the runners who would not participate in the walking and running protocol in the NaturalSport Cross-training Study at the USOTC was still in the back of my mind when I flew to St. Louis to meet with the management team of NaturalSport walking shoes.

Ever since Dr. Byrnes had informed me that he and Dr. Kearney could not get any runners to participate in their protocol at the USOTC, I had been dreaming of a way to smoke the runners out. I wanted a way to make them prove that they are better athletes than race walkers. In our meeting I laid out for the NaturalSport executives the details of what I believed would be one of the most widely watched, most challenging track biathlons ever held. In my proposal NaturalSport would contact organizers of national running events such as the Boston and New York City marathons to scour the United States for the two best male American runners. NaturalSport would do likewise to find the two best female race walkers. In a neutral location—perhaps the USOTC training center—the athletes would all train in their sports for 90 days, under strict surveillance to prohibit cross-training in the opposite sport.

A 10K (6.2-mile) race walk and 10K run biathlon would then

be held. This is the equivalent of a 20K (12.4 miles) event, or approximately a mini-marathon. The conditions of the race would be simple. The race walk would be judged so that each athlete truly race-walked. Each athlete would bring to the event the best conditioning possible for the gait he or she represented and would have to gut it out in the other gait without cross-training.

Since male runners wouldn't show up for free at the USOTC to cooperate in the cross-training protocol, the question now was, Would any of them show up for a chance to win $25,000 for competing against a *female*? NaturalSport would guarantee each male runner $25,000 if he won, and each female race walker $25,000 for winning. The reason for pitting a female walker against a male runner is that a male walker against a male runner probably would not be much of a contest. The male walker figures to win handily.

It is well established, however, that there is a male advantage of at least 10 to 15 percent over a female in track and field events. That's why men race men and women race women. In this race walk–run biathlon, the female race walker would actually be conceding a 10 to 15 percent advantage to the male runner before the starting gun even sounded. In addition, as pointed out earlier in this chapter, the pool of good female race walkers in the United States is small. There are far more champion-caliber male runners, which gives them a big talent edge.

I believed that this biathlon would draw one of the largest audiences of any non-Olympic track and field event in this century. There are over 71 million exercise walkers in this country and 23 million runners and joggers. Add to that the number of people who have a natural curiosity about a male-versus-female athletic contest (remember Billie Jean King and Bobby Riggs's tennis match?), and practically the whole country, as well as other countries, would tune in.

ABC's *Wide World of Sports* probably could not find a track event with greater audience potential. And, who knows, race walking might even get a mention in *USA Today*. The only remaining problem was finding two high-ranked male runners to take up the challenge.

The NaturalSport management team agreed that this would be a sporting event with enormous appeal. They promised me that NaturalSport would guarantee $25,000 prize money for each of the two race walk–run biathlon winners. Upon publication of this book, NaturalSport will contact organizers of running events to see if they can find champion-caliber runners to participate in the NaturalSport $50,000 Race Walk–Run Biathlon. We have tried to make the running proponents an offer they can't refuse: $50,000 in prize money, and male runners will get to race against female walkers. Any takers?

In the athletic contest I have proposed, you will notice I continually refer to gaits. In my view, this biathlon is more a contest between gaits than one between humans. As bipeds, we have mistakenly focused on running, our secondary gait, as being superior to walking not only as an exercise but as a sport. Runners have been lionized, glamorized, and idolized in this country. I believe it is time to penetrate the unwarranted aura of athletic superiority that runners have surrounded themselves with and see how the running gait stacks up against the walking gait–head to head and without cross-training!

Quite honestly, I have an ulterior motive in all this. First, as you know by now, I am convinced, and I hope you are too, that walking as an exercise and sport has been vastly underrated and underutilized in relation to running. In this biathlon, I feel confident that race walking, the ugly duckling of track and field events, will turn out to be a big, beautiful swan. This will be a spectacular opportunity to give walking instant parity with running, and maybe even nudge it ahead a little.

The thrust of this book is not to make race walkers out of people but to make exercisers out of them. When everyone sees how well the walking gait performs in this biathlon, the millions of people who don't like to run will realize that walking is truly the complete exercise. They will know it can be as effective as they want it to be—even superior to running. If I can influence people to get up and walk at whatever pace they will follow *consistently*, I know they will have made a major contribution to their health and longevity.

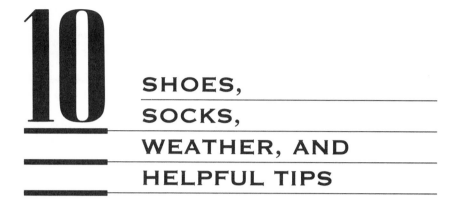

10

SHOES,
SOCKS,
WEATHER, AND
HELPFUL TIPS

SHOES

Not only did exercise walking have to launch itself, but there was even a time when the necessity of an exercise-walking shoe was in doubt. "Do Exercise Walkers Need Special Walking Shoes?" was a feature article in the June 1987 issue of *The Physician and Sportsmedicine* magazine. Out of nowhere, exercise walking had emerged and, as *The Physician and Sportsmedicine* reported, it was not until 1986 that the National Sporting Goods Association gathered the first statistics on it. In its initial walking-activities survey, the association projected 49.7 million exercise walkers, compared with an estimated 33.0 million joggers. The significance of this comparison is that jogging had been a popular, widely publicized aerobic exercise for over eight years; yet exercise walking, still in its infancy, had already taken the lead by a wide margin.

With such impressive numbers, the shoe manufacturers obviously had to get interested in exercise walking in a big way. They did, and by April 1991 *The Walking Magazine*, in its "Buyer's Guide" issue, reported on 57 models of exercise-walking shoes. In answer to its own question about the need for exercise-walking shoes, *The Physician and Sportsmedicine* quoted Sebastian Di

Casoli, director of marketing services for the Sporting Goods Manufacturing Association, who observed that there was no clear technical rationale for a walking-shoe design. He said, "Right now, the definition of a walking shoe is whatever anyone wants to make. . . . Some manufacturers have technical approaches, some are making clones of jogging shoes, and most are somewhere in between. The walking shoe is evolving as a category."

Unfortunately the evolution of the walking shoe has not been as clear-cut as that of the walking gait. In addition, many of the early walking "experts" advised that jogging shoes were good enough for walkers. Most of the big athletic shoe companies are involved primarily with the running gait, so they tended to make their version of the walking shoe a jogging-shoe clone.

Going back 3 million years to Lucy or 6,000 years to the Garden of Eden, the human foot has functioned quite well by walking and running without shoes. Even today in less-developed countries approximately 2 billion people spend their whole lives walking and running barefoot, or in nothing more than thong sandals. Empirical evidence indicates that they have fewer foot problems than those of us who wear shoes. In February 1986, the *University of California at Berkeley Wellness Letter* observed, "Ill-fitting shoes, it is thought, cause 80 percent of all foot problems. Besides causing corns, bunions, nail deformities, and other problems, painful shoes can alter your gait and your outlook for the worse."

Nevertheless, in Western industrialized countries we wear shoes, and there is a bewildering array of styles, colors, and models of athletic or exercise shoes to choose from. How do you choose the right one amidst all the marketing claims? A quick review of the differences between the biomechanics of the walking and running gaits will show you why a running shoe and some other models are counterproductive for an exercise walker.

Features of a Good Walking Shoe

As you know from Chapter 3, a runner is airborne on each step and hits the running surface with a force about 3.5 times his or her body weight. The body's entire mass is loaded abruptly onto a single foot. Humans were not biomechanically engineered with an effective shock-absorbing system, so the running-shoe companies have tried to devise one by strapping a collision mat to the bottom of the foot. They have come up with all kinds of ingenious devices—air bags, gels, and tubings—designed to mask the shock of running and supposedly reduce injuries.

For instance, back in the mid-1980s, one of the early ads for the then new Nike Air Cushion Shoe showed an automobile crash test with an air bag deployed. The ad copy stated: "On average, you'll crash 17,600 times during a 10-mile trip. And with every single impact, shock waves will be sent tearing through your body at speeds up to 120 miles-per-hour. We're talking about running. And the most important reason you need Nike—air cushioning." Does anybody, by the wildest stretch of the imagination, believe that a little air bag on the bottom of your foot could effectively absorb or dissipate much shock to your musculoskeletal system?

Essentially, in the shoe companies' minds, a running shoe is designed for "Damage Control." That was the main theme of Etonic's ad campaign for its new running shoe in the April 1991 "Spring Shoe Buyer's Guide" of *Runner's World*. The first line of the ad read, "The damage report is in; 61.6% of all runners were injured last year." It is obvious that the air bags, gels, and other gimmicks cannot overcome the basic fact that the human animal is not designed for frequent, prolonged running.

The big, thick heel and squishy sole that act as a collision mat in Figure 10.1, which shows a generic-type running shoe, are counterproductive for the walking gait, and, in spite of marketing claims, they also don't seem to be effective in preventing running injuries. The walking gait lets the walker load his or her body weight onto the foot in a nonimpact, gentle way. A walker does not need a defensive shoe, designed to absorb impact, but an offensive shoe that will permit the foot to function naturally in its most biomechanically efficient manner. In effect, an exercise-walking shoe's design should be exactly the opposite of a running shoe.

People buy dress shoes primarily because of the quality of leather, color, texture, and decorative design of their uppers (the top part of the shoe). In an exercise-walking shoe, however, it's what's under the foot that's more important. The way the walking platform of a shoe is designed from the heel, where the walking motion begins, to the toe, where the foot must bend for toe-off, determines how your foot will function. Anything that inhibits the natural motion of the foot, which functioned without shoes or

FIGURE 10.1

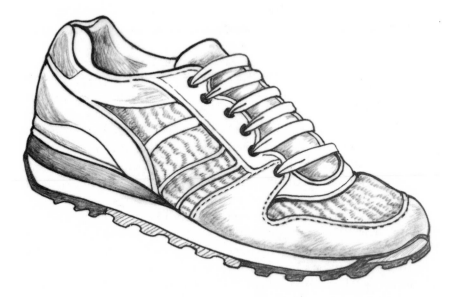

sandals until recent times, will affect the foot's biomechanical efficiency. In other words, your foot and the muscles in your legs will be fighting the restrictions of the shoe.

Heel elevation is a prime consideration in the walking motion. Dr. Inman observes that women in high heels take shorter steps than do women in low heels. When I do a walking clinic for NaturalSport walking shoes, I always ask the women what they do with their high-heeled dress shoes when they get home from church or a party? In unison they sing out, "Take 'em off!" The obvious reason, of course, is to get the heel back down where it belongs, in its most natural position.

The primary role of the walking platform is to protect the bottom of the foot. This role has not changed since the first sandal was made several thousand years ago. In addition, the walking platform must provide moderate cushioning for comfort on our hard walking surfaces. Remember, there were no concrete, asphalt, or macadam roads until recent times. The evolution of the walking gait occurred on terra firma.

A good walking-shoe platform should provide adequate protection and the proper amount of cushioning without elevating the heel too far from its natural position, which distorts the walking motion. It is nearly impossible to get the right combination of cushioning and protection in a walking platform that is less than ½-inch thick at the heel. It is also apparent that, when the heel is elevated beyond ¾ inch, it starts to alter the biomechanical efficiency of the foot. Therefore, the best range of heel heights for walking shoes is ½ to ¾ inch. I prefer a heel closer to ½ inch, because I like to walk fast, and it is easier to do so in a lower heel.

Overbuilt heels are one of the major reasons running shoes are not good walking shoes. Another reason is that running shoes are too soft at the heel for a walker. When a walker loads his or her weight onto a running shoe's high, squishy heel, it continues to compress as the walker's weight comes down on the foot. This is a microversion of walking on sand. When you walk on the beach and your foot continues to sink as you load your weight on it, you quickly get tired leg muscles. Trying to walk fast in running shoes causes a similar fatigue. Admittedly you can walk slowly in any kind of shoes—or with no shoes at all. A good walking shoe, however, should permit you to walk efficiently at the low, moderate, and high-intensity levels.

One of the early makers of exercise-walking shoes (I will not mention it by name) designed a walking platform that was about 1 inch high at the heel and rigid from the heel to the toe. The company called it a "rocker" design, and it was supposed to aid the walking motion. It sent me a pair. These are comfortable shoes at a slow stroll, but as you attempt the brisk pace the rigid forefoot of the walking platform fights the natural bending movement of the foot at toe-off and causes fatigue in the legs. It is like putting a governor on your foot; you cannot walk faster than a 15-minute mile without considerable leg stress.

A good walking-shoe platform should not be rigid at the forefoot (the ball of the foot), as many jogging and "cross-trainer" shoes are. Each foot has 26 bones, approximately 56 ligaments, and 38 muscles. It is a complex piece of biomechanical work. The ability of all those bones, ligaments, and muscles to function naturally and without impediment is essential to the walking motion. Rigid soles at the forefoot on exercise-walking shoes interfere with toe-off, which is an essential part of the foot's contribution to your forward progress.

Dr. Inman's research in *Human Walking* addresses the way the foot reacts biomechanically from heel plant to toe-off. In his sum-

FIGURE 10.2A   **FIGURE 10.2B**

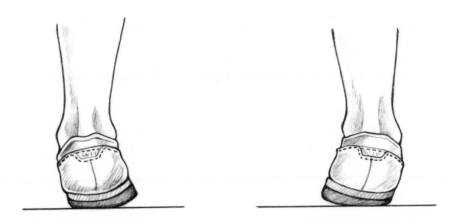

mary, he states: "As the foot is loaded, it can be seen to pronate. As the heel is raised, there is a rapid but slight inversion of the heel as the foot supinates." The terms *pronate* and *supinate* are better understood visually than by a lengthy definition. Figure 10.2A shows a *pronating* foot, and Figure 10.2B shows a *supinating* foot.

If you are at home, you can see how your foot reacts when you load your weight onto it. Take your shoe and sock off one foot. With your foot slightly in front of you and your toes up, as if you were taking a short step, place your heel on the floor, slowly lower your forefoot onto the floor, and bring your body over it. As your forefoot comes down so that all your weight is evenly distributed on the whole foot, you will notice that your medial ankle area will bulge slightly and tend to roll to the inside (pronate). On most overweight or obese people, these tendencies are quite pronounced.

As you load your weight onto your forefoot and toes, notice how your forefoot widens and the middle toes tend to spread. When your heel rises as you start to toe off, observe how your foot shifts to the outside edge (supinates) as you transfer all your weight to the front of it. When the forefoot is in the last stages of flexing before toe-off, you will notice that it bends at an oblique angle just behind the toes.

Dr. Inman calls this oblique angle between the toes and meta-

FIGURE 10.3

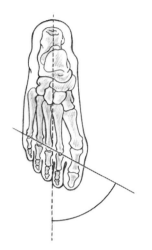

tarsal bones the "metatarsophalangeal break" (pronounced met a tar´so fa lan´je al). The metatarsals are the big bones in the forefoot to which the phalanges (toes) are connected. Figure 10.3 shows the metatarsophalangeal angle in relation to the long axis of the foot. Dr. Inman points out: "To distribute the weight between all metatarsal heads, the foot must deviate laterally (supinate) at push-off."

Supple forefoot flex in an exercise-walking shoe is absolutely essential to accommodate the foot's natural break at toe-off, as shown in Figure 10.3. Some "rocker"-type shoes, most cross-trainers, and jogging shoes are too rigid at this critical biomechanical juncture. They restrict the foot's ability to contribute to forward propulsion at toe-off and cause the foot to labor against the stiff walking platform as it tries to bend in its natural manner. A walker wearing such shoes and trying to accelerate beyond the brisk pace will experience unnecessary shin fatigue and stress in the leg muscles.

A good walking shoe should have a stiff pronation support band called a heel counter around the medial side and back of the shoe, at the point where the upper joins the walking platform. In addition, a walking shoe should have a wide toe box to accommodate the widening of the forefoot when the body weight is loaded onto

FIGURE 10.4

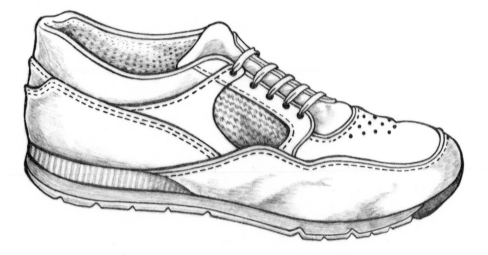

it. The toe box should also be high enough to give the toes adequate clearance. Figure 10.4 shows a generic walking shoe.

The platform of an exercise-walking shoe should be essentially neutral. It should not try to manage the foot's biomechanics but should let it move from heel plant to toe-off in its most natural manner. It should be thick enough (but no thicker than ¾ inch at the heel) to protect the bottom of the foot, and provide a moderate amount of cushioning. Shoe manufacturers who claim they have a "walking system that propels your foot forward" probably have Sir Isaac Newton spinning in his grave. Once you load your weight onto your front foot, the only thing that will propel you forward is your hind foot as you push off.

A variety of materials and constructions are used in exercise-walking-shoe platforms. The most common combination is a molded platform consisting of a rubber "outsole" that makes contact with the walking surface. A "midsole" is a cushioning material sandwiched between the outsole and the "insole," which is what the foot rests on inside the shoe.

The uppers should be made of breathable leather or a nylon mesh–leather combination. Good walking shoes have removable insole inserts that have a built-up arch control. These inserts can be removed to dry if wet from sweat. Most people like a shoe with significant support in the arch area, but some do not. Remember the millions of people on the planet right now who walk barefoot or in thong sandals their whole life with no arch support.

How to Buy Walking Shoes

When you go shopping for exercise-walking shoes, do not assume the shoe clerk knows anything about walking as an exercise or how an exercise-walking shoe should differ from a jogging shoe. Most salespeople in athletic shoe stores are more familiar with running and are not knowledgeable about exercise walking. I have yet to find one who was. They are likely to recommend a walking shoe made by a major athletic-shoe company simply because they have sold the company's running shoes and are familiar with the brand name. You may be getting a jogging shoe clone. You must be your own walking-shoe expert and know what to look for.

Now I will give you the sequence to follow to buy the most important piece of equipment an exercise walker needs: properly fitting walking shoes. Your buying decision should always be made on the basis of *fit and comfort* over any technical features. If the shoes don't fit right and feel good on your feet the moment you put them on, you won't be a happy walker. There is no break-in period for walking shoes!

Here is the buying sequence to follow:

1. It is best to buy shoes at midday, or after you have had your daily walk. Feet may swell up to a half size over the course of the day.

2. Always fit shoes wearing the kind of socks you walk in. Women should not fit exercise-walking shoes in hose unless they walk in them. (I have known some older women who do.)

3. Get both feet measured with the measuring device that shoe stores use every time you buy shoes. Foot size can change, particularly if you have gained or lost a lot of weight.

4. Always stand and load your weight onto the foot being measured. Your forefoot widens when it is bearing weight.

5. Put both shoes on and lace them up evenly. Some clerks leave the lower laces loose and merely snug them at the top eyelets. You want to know how the upper forms to your entire foot and how

it holds the walking platform in place. Take an extra 10 seconds and lace the shoes up evenly and snugly.

6. *This is critical: check the shoes on a hard surface.* Department stores have a hard-surface aisle, and shopping malls are hard surfaced outside the shoe store. Most people stand around on carpet trying to make a buying decision. They end up looking in the little mirror down on the floor to see if the shoes look attractive on their feet and buy them more for cosmetic reasons than for biomechanical functionality.

7. On a hard surface, walk 10 or 15 steps at your fastest pace; do so back and forth several times. Check how your weight is loaded onto the foot at heel plant and how your foot rolls forward to toe-off. Is the shoe flexible in the forefoot? Is there rubbing or tightness anywhere? Is the toe box wide enough? Is there looseness at the heel? Walking at *your* fastest pace lets your foot interact with the shoe and the walking surface to bring out any deficiencies. Most shoes feel pretty good when you are standing on a carpet or just taking a few slow steps. The acid test for a walking shoe is to put your foot in action on a hard surface, just as you do on your daily walk. I recommend that you walk-check regular dress shoes the same way. You'll be surprised how quickly you can eliminate ill-fitting shoes before buying them.

8. Many people have one foot a bit longer than the other. Always accommodate the longer foot when sizing. About ¼- to ½-inch clearance should be allowed between your toe and the end of the toe box. If you walk-check the shoe thoroughly, you will find out at toe-off whether you have adequate clearance.

9. Don't hesitate to try on several brands. If one feels good, another might feel even better. Buy a walking shoe that comes in actual width sizes. Most good walking shoes are made on at least four lasts: narrow, medium, wide, and double wide. As a rule, jogging shoes are made only on a medium last.

10. Examine the heel area carefully. Do not buy a walking shoe that doesn't have a good, strong heel counter for pronation control. This is particularly important if you are overweight.

11. Check the forefoot area for flex. Can you take the shoe in your hand and easily bend it to the angle at which your foot naturally bends at toe-off? If not, the shoe will fight your foot as you try to walk at the brisk pace or faster.

An exception to this rule is a hiking shoe. Of necessity it will have a stiffer, thicker sole for protection of the foot in off-pavement walking. Hiking is much slower than brisk-paced walking, and the toe-off is minimal. The theoretical exercise-walking shoe described earlier was meant for low-, moderate-, and high-intensity exercise walking on smooth, paved surfaces. A shoe that functions well on this kind of surface will lack the protection and rigidity for walking on uneven, off-pavement surfaces. If you hike, you should have hiking shoes that can accommodate those conditions.

12. A good exercise-walking shoe should be light, preferably weighing less than 11 ounces.

Buying the lowest-priced shoe may cause you to pay a higher price later in foot and other problems. At 1991 prices, a good pair of exercise-walking shoes will cost between $55 and $80. National discount stores advertise athletic-looking shoes for $30 or less, but they have cheap composition material in the midsoles that mashes down and often aggravates pronation.

In a clinic in the spring of 1990, a middle-aged woman told me she was starting to have knee and back discomfort after her daily walks in a large shopping mall. I looked at her shoes. They weren't worn out; in fact, they looked as if they had just come out of the box. They had a generic look, and I didn't recognize them by make. I asked her where she'd gotten them, how long she'd had them, and how much she'd paid for them. She had bought them from one of the leading discount stores, had had them eight weeks, and proudly proclaimed that they cost only $23. Her discomfort had started about three weeks after buying those shoes.

I got behind her and asked her to walk away from me at her fastest pace. In only a few steps, I could see that she was pronating badly as she loaded her weight onto her foot at heel plant. I then had her take both shoes off and walk away from me again. She hardly pronated at all when barefoot. The midsoles of her shoes had mashed down on the medial side, creating a situation like a slanted sidewalk, so that every time she took a step her foot came down in an exaggerated, slanted position. The shoe thus sent stress and torque up her leg.

As a word of caution, all athletic-type shoes look pretty good when brand-new. The difference between a $25 pair and a $65 pair is in the materials, construction, and support systems. Remember, you only get what you pay for. Don't buy cheap athletic-type shoes for exercise walking!

Finally, most people keep their shoes too long. Internal wear and compression are not always obvious. Midsoles compress with the constant loading of the body weight, reducing the cushioning effect. Shoes also stretch sometimes, altering their support. One way to tell if you need new shoes is to have someone watch you walk from behind. If your feet are pronating more in the shoes than when you walk barefoot, get rid of them. Remember that a good pair of walking shoes is not an expense but an investment in your health and happiness.

A PODIATRIST MAY BE YOUR BEST FRIEND

No other part of the body is more biomechanically complex and works harder under extreme loads than the foot. We all tend to look down at the tops of our shoes and assume that the foot is a monolithic lump. Inside those shoes, however, are mazes of bones, ligaments, and muscles that must interact smoothly and efficiently at each step.

For advice about the foot, I sought out Dr. Howard Palamarchuk, who is on the faculty at the Pennsylvania College of Podiatric Medicine in Philadelphia. He is the director of sports medicine and clinical instructor in orthopedics. I particularly wanted Dr. Palamarchuk's input because he has observed the foot under the most extreme, stressful conditions since he is the sports medicine chairman for race walking at The Athletic Congress. In addition, he was a race walker and tried out for the Olympics in 1972. He knows from personal experience how much punishment the feet can take.

Even though the walking gait is injury free, many people in this country and other Western industrialized countries experience foot problems when they take up exercise walking. Some of these problems can be eliminated before they start; others can be managed with the help of a good podiatrist.

Dr. Palamarchuk says that the most common foot problem he sees in exercise walkers, particularly beginning walkers, is overuse. The foot of a sedentary person, like the rest of his body, is unfit. Many people abruptly start a walking program and activate the foot without gradually getting it into condition.

The 2 billion people who walk barefoot or in sandals use the walking gait as their primary form of locomotion. From their first steps as children to their graves, their feet are used constantly, day in and day out, mile after mile. They become fit and tough and stay that way through their entire lives. Soft, sedentary people in

Western industrialized countries spend most of their lives sitting or riding. For many, the foot has lost its strength and durability, much like an arm or leg that has been in a cast.

Most problems occur, however, because of poor equipment, according to Dr. Palamarchuk. He believes that people, particularly those who are overweight or those who tend to pronate, make a major mistake by walking in cheap shoes.

In the spring of 1990, when I traveled coast-to-coast for NaturalSport introducing their new Aerobic Walker shoe, I became aware of the great number of people who have foot problems. Bunions, heel spurs, and hammertoes can make life miserable for a walker, yet, with the help of a good podiatrist, most of these situations can be managed successfully. Carol had both feet operated on for extremely painful bunions ten years ago. Today she can do the triple nickel at 52 years of age.

Dr. Palamarchuk believes that heel spurs are caused by bad shoes more than anything else and also that "pronation contributes to them." He points out that many people have benign, asymptomatic heel spurs for years and don't know it. When they start walking a lot of miles in nonsupportive, poorly constructed shoes, the heel spurs become painful. Once this occurs, good shoes won't help until the pain is dissipated, usually with rest and ice. For some, the condition requires a trip to the podiatrist.

Managing foot problems sometimes requires an orthotic. A podiatrist can build a molded bed for your foot that gives it constant support and balance where it is needed. This slips inside the shoe. I know many exercise walkers who have traveled a lot of happy miles on their orthotics. Without them they don't walk far without considerable discomfort. Dr. Palamarchuk says, "There are few foot problems that can't be solved, or at least successfully controlled, with today's state-of-the-art podiatry." If you experience nagging foot problems when you take up exercise walking, I suggest you have a good podiatrist check your feet and walking shoes.

One final comment on walking shoes. I have made it very clear that I am the walking consultant for NaturalSport. Walking shoes are the only kind of exercise shoes this company makes. Their Aerobic Walker has all the technical features that a good exercise-walking shoe should have to take you through the low-, moderate-, and high-intensity levels of walking. I recommend that you try them, along with several other brands, when you buy your next pair. *Walk-check them all*; then make your buying decision on the basis of fit, comfort, heel stability, forefoot flex, and the overall walking action of the shoe. Let your feet tell you which shoe to buy.

SOCKS

I have on my desk an ad for a major brand of athletic sock that says it is "cushion-engineered." A picture of the sock has arrows pointing to the heel and forefoot, accompanied by this copy, "Heavyweight Plus cushioning across the sole protects the heel and ball against concussion and shock." If you buy this line, the Brooklyn Bridge can also be yours for a sawbuck. How much concussion and shock can a little bit of yarn on the bottom of your foot absorb?

The role of the sock is to provide an environment between your foot and the shoe. If you have proper shoes, they will take care of all the cushioning you need. Besides, concussion and shock are not a problem for walkers. A smooth-fitting sock that conforms to your foot and doesn't wrinkle is all you need. Wrinkles in a sock will rub your foot and cause blisters. I have acquired more blisters from socks than I have from shoes. Do not buy "tube-type" socks. The worst case of blisters I ever had came from a discount store bargain on tube socks—"6 pairs for 6 bucks." I began to get blisters under my middle toes. It took me three weeks to figure out that the material of the ill-fitting tube socks was gathering under my toes and rubbing when I toed off.

When the exercise-walking movement got big, the sock companies who had been wooing runners saw a larger market and immediately invented "walking socks." But the "engineering" in walking socks is advertising hype. If the sock is your size and form-fitting, wear it.

Cotton socks absorb moisture and lose their shape when wet. This can cause wrinkles and blisters. There are a number of synthetic materials that "wick" moisture away from the foot, and I prefer these to cotton or wool. For the past four years I have worn Double Lay-R socks, made with DuPont Cool Max fiber for warm weather and DuPont Thermax fiber for cold weather. They are double-layer socks but don't feel like it because they aren't bulky. They come with a money-back or replacement guarantee if you experience blisters or the socks wear out within 1,000 miles. I have a couple of pairs that must have 5,000 miles on them. Double Lay-

R socks are sold in most major and independent athletic shoe stores. However, if the socks you are wearing are not causing you blisters and you are pleased with them, there is no need to change.

CLOTHING

It seems as if all the jazzy, good-looking athletic clothing was designed for runners and aerobic classes. Most of the early walking outfits bordered on sackcloth and ashes; walkers were supposed to look dowdy. Maybe those days are over. In the spring of 1991, a new catalog arrived called "Walk USA." (You can get a copy by calling 1-800-255-6422.) It had bright colors, walking tights, good-looking shorts, and a wide variety of walking shoes, socks, and fanny packs—just about anything a woman walker needs.

The catalog was aimed at women walkers, but that's all right—since they represent about two thirds of the walking population. Carol bought a couple of pairs of the brightly colored tights and looks terrific in them. Walkers should wear athletic clothes as upbeat and colorful as runners do. We are as athletic and fit as they are. I buy fleeced and unfleeced sweatpants and shirts, as well as walking shorts from L. L. Bean in bright colors. A number of catalogs are now featuring good-looking walking apparel.

Walking clothing should be comfortable and nonbinding in the legs, arms, and shoulders. Jeans are too restrictive and do not permit the legs enough freedom. Women probably should not exercise-walk in skirts. Even a wide skirt bumping the front of the leg tends to inhibit a good, fast stride. I consider my daily walk a workout, and the clothes I wear are the athletic type rather than an old pair of pants. Sweats and shorts don't cost much and last a long time. Having workout gear is as appropriate for a walker as it is for a runner. Dress athletically and you'll feel athletic, no matter how old you are.

WEATHER: HOT AND COLD

Exercise walking in hot weather can be treacherous, especially for an older, out-of-shape person. Don't go out in the midday hours if the temperature reaches 90 degrees and above; it can be dangerous. Don't worry about aerobic speed, and shorten your walk if you feel light-headed or dizzy. When we have those July–August Missouri heat waves, I generally walk at 6:00 A.M. Even then the combination of heat and humidity makes it difficult to breathe easily. You'll find that such weather makes your legs seem heavy and hard to move; it will test your resolve. As long as you protect yourself against sunstroke and dehydration, however, there is no reason not to walk. You don't have to push as hard or walk as far, but don't give up your routine.

Once in a while in hot weather, I start out slowly (a 15-minute-mile pace) and decide to just poke along. By the second or third mile, when I'm wringing with sweat, something seems to break loose, and I finish as strongly as if it were a cool day. Your body will tell you when to go fast and when to coast. Don't assume that you have to hit top speed every day in hot weather, but also don't assume that you can't hit top speed on a hot day. Listen to your body.

Drink plenty of water before you start out and plenty when you come back. Most of us don't drink enough water. Doctors recommend six to eight glasses a day. If you walk aerobically for 30 minutes to an hour each day in hot weather, be sure you drink this much. You'll need it.

Cold weather is the other extreme to be faced in many parts of the country. As people get older, their tolerance for cold seems to diminish; that's why the Sunbelt is such a popular retirement area. For those who don't mind it, cold-weather walking can be the most invigorating and enjoyable of all, but you must dress properly for it. The most dangerous aspect of cold weather for a walker is not low temperature, but wind. A windchill of 5 degrees or more below zero is something to fear. Even proper clothing can't produce a comfort level at which you can walk with smooth biomechanical movements when it's frigid out. Leg muscles take forever to warm up, and on some days they never do.

Table 10.1 is a windchill index. Dr. Neil Gordon advises that a windchill below 15° F is not recommended for cardiac patients. All TV stations announce windchills in the winter, and in some ways they are more important than actual temperature. You will find that a light wind of 5 miles per hour and a cold temperature is easier to tolerate and less chilling than a high wind of 20 miles per hour and slightly warmer temperatures.

On a cold, windy day, the most important rule to remember is *always start your walk headed into the wind.* Doing so is uncomfortable, but it will tell you right away whether it is too cold to walk at all. You won't walk far before you'll know if this is a day

TABLE 10.1.

Windchill index

WIND SPEED (mph)	AMBIENT TEMPERATURE (°F)								
	50	40	30	20	10	0	−10	−20	−30
	Windchill Index (°F)								
Calm	50	40	30	20	10	0	−10	−20	−30
5	48	37	27	16	6	−5	−15	−26	−36
10	40	28	16	4	−9	−21	−33	−46	−58
15	36	22	9	−5	−18	−36	−45	−58	−72
20	32	18	4	−10	−25	−39	−53	−67	−82
25	30	16	0	−15	−29	−44	−59	−74	−88
30	28	13	−2	−18	−33	−48	−63	−79	−94
35	27	11	−4	−20	−35	−49	−67	−82	−98
40	26	10	−6	−21	−37	−53	−69	−85	−100

When the windchill index falls below 15°F, outdoor exercise is not recommended for cardiac patients.
SOURCE: Neil F. Gordon, M.D., and Larry W. Gibbons, M.D., *The Cooper Clinic Cardiac Rehabilitation Program.* New York: Simon & Schuster, 1990.

when you should just pack it in. If you start out with your back to the wind, you can be a couple of miles from home before you realize that the return trip is unbearable, and by then you're in trouble. Frostbite can occur quickly. The other negative about wind, particularly gusty wind, is the natural tendency to lean into it. This will throw your erect posture off, and you'll tire your back and shoulder muscles. Even on days when the windchill is not a factor, wind can louse up your walk because it affects your posture. Cold-weather walking without wind, however, is a delight.

Cold-weather clothing should be worn in layers. It is better to overdress so that you can peel off a layer or two than to be shivering and wishing you had worn more. It is impossible to walk with the proper posture if you are cold, especially if you're feeling the chill in the chest and rib cage. For walking in temperatures below 25 degrees, an essential piece of clothing is an insulated vest. The L. L. Bean catalog or stores such as K mart, J. C. Penney, and Sears all carry them. You don't need an expensive goose-down vest; an inexpensive synthetic one works fine. The rest of your clothing can be standard-brand thermal long-john tops and bottoms, cotton turtleneck shirts, sweatpants, a nylon windbreaker, a cap with ear flaps or a stocking cap, and warm gloves or mittens.

Some people have a greater tolerance for cold than others, so you'll have to experiment with how many layers you need at 20, 10, and 0 degrees. Below zero, forget it. Keep your eye on the temperature and windchill. When in doubt, wear more, not less. Stepping out the front door to test the weather is not a good gauge. You will be tempted to think it is not as cold as it really is because you are still warm, and a few seconds outside won't give you a good indication of what to expect. Put your nylon windbreaker on over your vest. As you heat up, you can peel it off first and tie it around your waist. You are then in a position to open your vest and let air in around your rib cage if you become really hot. Cold weather helps you burn more calories, which is an added reason to get outside for your walk. It also makes you step right along, and the faster you walk, the warmer you stay.

In cold weather many people make the mistake of walking with their hands jammed in the pockets of their jackets. It is important to have your arms loose and swinging freely to counterbalance your leg swing. Insulated gloves or mittens will keep your hands warm. Cold weather invites fast walking, and if your arms are neutralized, your ability to walk fast in a smooth, rhythmic manner is reduced. You also eliminate the activity of the major muscle groups in the chest, shoulders, and back, which contributes to your caloric expenditure and overall fitness.

RULES OF THE ROAD AND SAFETY TIPS

I walk on two-lane country roads where there are no sidewalks. A cardinal rule for anyone who walks on a road is *always walk facing the traffic*. Other rules of the road are

1. Even though you may have the right-of-way at an intersection, make eye contact with the driver of an approaching car so that he or she will acknowledge your presence.

2. Always look both ways before crossing a street or intersection.

3. Stay on the outside of a blind curve if the road is narrow.

4. On two-lane roads, step onto the shoulder to allow oncoming

cars to pass if one is coming from the other direction. It's the courteous thing to do.

5. For walking at twilight or at night, always wear reflective strips on your clothing.

6. Wear white or bright-colored clothing on gray, cloudy days.

Those of us who live in the serenity of a rural area only have to worry about the dangers of automobiles. Unfortunately, people living in many areas of large cities also have to think about personal safety. Here are some guidelines to follow in that regard:

1. Try to find a walking buddy, especially if you are a woman.

2. Know the area where you are walking and any businesses that will be open during your walk. Stay out of isolated areas.

3. If possible, walk when there is other pedestrian traffic.

4. Don't walk at night in unlit, isolated areas.

5. Vary your walks so that you don't have a set routine.

6. When walking in parks, stay away from dense brush and wooded areas.

7. Don't walk close to doorways or courtyards.

8. Let someone know where you are going and when you expect to be back.

9. Women should carry a police whistle and a can of Mace in their fanny packs.

10. Don't wear jewelry. Carry a dollar's worth of change for phone calls if needed.

11. Carry an identification tag in your pocket or fanny pack with your name, address, phone number, and blood type.

12. If you are wearing a Walkman or headphones, scan the area around you constantly, even glancing backward once in a while. Walk defensively because you may not hear someone coming from the rear.

These personal safety guidelines were difficult for me to write. Sadly, in all of the animal kingdom, the human animal can be the most vicious and unpredictable. I would not trade the country roads I share with rabbits, squirrels, coyotes, deer, and a mix of farm dogs for any city street and the human danger that goes with it.

MALL WALKING

Shopping malls have become a great asset to the exercise-walking movement. Many people walk in them to escape the hazards of city streets. Others like their predictable climate. I have conducted walking clinics in almost a hundred major shopping malls, and many people tell me they wouldn't walk at all if they couldn't do so in a mall.

In the northern tier states, people escape harsh winter weather in malls. In the South, particularly in cities like Houston and New Orleans, which have heat coupled with high humidity, malls are comfortable too. The average age of mall walkers is about 60, so climatic conditions and personal safety are major concerns for them. If you are just starting a walking program and want to walk where the action is, check out a mall near you.

The shopping mall in St. Joseph, Missouri, near where I live, is typical of many that cater to "mall walkers." It opens at 6:00 A.M. to let walkers get an early start. One and a half trips around the perimeter is about a mile. Many of the regular walkers do 5 miles a day. Some walk at a 15-minute-mile pace, but most of them stroll.

Most people at the St. Joseph mall say they are walking for their health and to lose weight. One woman said she has lost 51 pounds by walking. Quite a few people have had heart problems. One 68-year-old widower said he likes the opportunity to meet people and has made over a hundred new acquaintances by walking at the mall. There is a certain camaraderie among mall walkers, especially the early birds. The stores don't open until 10:00 A.M., but all the hard-core walkers are there well before 7:00.

A shopping mall can be a good place for you to start walking. You will be exposed to others who have discovered the miracle of walking. You will hear health-improvement and weight-loss stories that will motivate you. Bear in mind that most mall walkers are fighting the same weight and fitness problems you have. You will find it easy to relate to them. Having twenty or thirty people with similar problems giving you encouragement to walk every day may mean more to you than anything you read in this book.

If you decide to walk in a mall, here are a couple of tips. Most people drive to a mall, and women usually bring a purse for their car keys. But carrying a purse or wearing a shoulder bag inhibits free arm swing. Get a small fanny pack to carry your wallet and car keys so that you can walk with vigor and a full arm swing. Practically everybody walks every little nook and cranny around the mall's perimeter, which means making too many short turns. This interrupts the pace and rhythm of the walk. Many malls are a quarter of a mile long. Pick the longest straightaway for your walk so that you can sustain a good, strong pace with few turns. A ¼-mile mall, for instance, would permit you to do ½ mile with only one turn. Walk the perimeter for your cool down, when pace is not important. If it is a nice day, try walking the perimeter of the mall's parking lot.

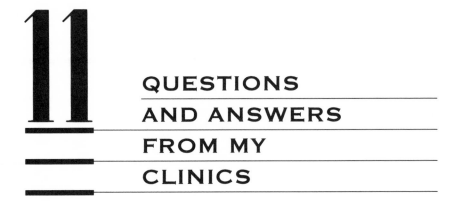

11

QUESTIONS
AND ANSWERS
FROM MY
CLINICS

My knowledge of walking and exercise is the result of continuous reading and research. From Dr. Lovejoy to Dr. Inman and all the others I have quoted, I have tried to be careful to select only sources that are scientifically correct. By the time you have reached this chapter, you probably have a pretty good idea of how your walking gait came about and how it works biomechanically.

The answers I give in the question-and-answer parts of my lectures sometimes are my own opinion, but most often they are the results of reading and research. I have answered many questions already, but the following are some others that are asked regularly. Many require detailed explanations. A few involve subjects on which there are widely differing opinions. Let's start with one of those.

Question: *What do you think of hand weights and ankle weights?*

Answer: Next to an ill-fitting pair of shoes, I can't think of anything that can ruin your walk quicker than hand or ankle weights. Using them is a dumb idea that just won't die, but I'll try one more time to kill it. The recommended use of weights for walkers is kept alive by sources that people assume are reliable. For instance, just before I started this chapter, an encyclopedia on wellness, health, and illness prevention that I ordered from one of the finest universities in the United States arrived. I checked the section entitled "Tips and Techniques for a Walking Program." Sure enough, there were those ubiquitous weights. The encyclopedia said, "As you get used to walking, carry a six-pound backpack or hand weights. You can substitute a briefcase or shopping bag for the backpack." How would you like to go out for a 3-mile exercise walk every day carrying a shopping bag or briefcase? How could you swing your arms?

Follow the science and rationale behind my answer, and let common sense be your guide.

Let's first pose the question, Why are weights recommended for walkers in the first place? The only reason is the assumption that they are needed to add *intensity* to the walking gait. But adding weights to walkers to achieve exercise intensity is as outdated as leisure suits. In Chapter 6 you learned to pick up the pace of your walk simply by swinging your arms faster with the bent-arm technique and by teaching your leg muscles to fire faster. The assumption that exercise walking lacks the intensity to be aerobic is without merit.

Weights aren't added to cyclists; they are told to pedal faster if they want exercise intensity. Weights aren't added to cross-country skiers; they just ski faster. You never see well-informed, knowledgeable runners carrying weights. Everyone assumes that these exercises are intensive enough to be aerobic, but so is walking if it is done properly.

Many of you reading this book are taking up walking for weight control, and the companies who sell weights often make outrageous and unfounded claims about how many extra calories they will help you burn. The July 1989 issue of the *Tufts University Diet and Nutrition Letter* cited a caloric expenditure study involving walkers with weights. It reported, "When eleven overweight people at the University of Missouri walked briskly with one-pound hand weights for a full thirty minutes, they burned only about 12 more calories than they did without the weights—a couple of Life Savers worth."

Dr. Harvey B. Simon, assistant professor of medicine at Harvard Medical School, gave some additional unimpressive caloric numbers in the September–October 1989 issue of *The Walking Mag-*

azine: "A 135 pound woman who walks vigorously can expect to burn about 200 calories in thirty minutes. Add 10 pounds of weights and you can expect to burn about 10 calories more. . . . You would have to carry those weights for about 300 miles to drop just one extra pound because of [them]. For comparison, walking itself will have taken off 30 pounds by then."

Walking should be a smooth, fluid, natural exercise. Biomechanically your arms and legs are properly balanced and should swing freely. Any weight you add to the ankles or hands unbalances your limbs and alters their normal swing for the worse, possibly even to the point of causing injury. Ankle weights can hyperextend your knees, and weights in general ruin your walk. Your object is to get the arm and leg pendulums swinging faster, and you can't do so by adding weights. On a risk-reward basis there are few things a walker could do that would be more counterproductive.

Question: *I live where there are hills. Will I burn a lot more calories walking uphill?*

Answer: A few nice, rolling hills add variety to a walk and may or may not burn a few extra calories. I often read articles in which a walker is advised that he or she can burn more calories by walking up hills. That's true, but the writers blithely seem to assume that there is one continuous hill. How about the return downhill? Without my getting into a deep technical explanation of "positive work" and "negative work," you already know that it is easier to walk down a hill or downstairs than it is to walk up. Gravity is pulling against you going up and pulling you toward your line of travel going down. Up is positive work, and down is negative work. That's a bit oversimplified, but you get the point.

If you walk up a hill, as I do every day, you have to walk down the other side, which burns fewer calories than walking up or walking on the level. A few days a month I wear a heart-rate monitor. It is interesting to observe how quickly my heart rate goes up when I'm climbing a hill, even though my pace slows, and how quickly it starts to drop as I crest the hill and head down the other side. I have to increase my speed considerably to keep my heart rate up when walking downhill, and so will you. If you average the up-and-down caloric expenditure of walking on hills, it may not be much better than that of a fast, sustainable pace on level ground.

FIGURE 11.1

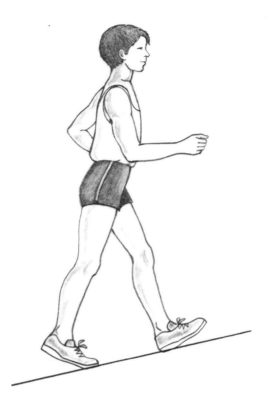

Question: *Is there a particular way to walk uphill or downhill?*
Answer: Going uphill, one's first inclination is to bend at the waist and lean into the hill. That's wrong, and if you do so you will soon have lower-back muscles that are fatigued and hurting. Leonard Jansen, the former race-walking analyst at the United States Olympic Training Center, advises that you should maintain proper erect posture and *shorten your stride* walking up a hill (see Figure 11.1).

Your pace will slow but the pull of gravity as you go uphill will make you work harder, and your heart rate will actually increase. Remember that, when you walk up stairs, the average stair riser is only about 8 inches high, so your step is automatically shortened. Keep your head up, your back straight from your ears to your ankles, and your shoulders over your hips. You can lean forward slightly by bending at the ankles, as race walkers do, but don't lose your posture. If the hill is extremely steep, like those in San Francisco, forget speed altogether and walk up it with the best posture possible. I also recommend that you find another place to walk. Hills like that create more posture problems than they are worth and are not enjoyable for exercise walking.

Walking downhill presents a different challenge. It is easy to keep your posture, but how do you increase speed to keep your heart rate up without jarring yourself senseless? Walking or running downhill is never as comfortable as walking on the level or uphill. There are two ways to walk downhill: (1) vertical to the line of gravity; (2) perpendicular to the slope of the hill. Leonard Jansen teaches both ways but advises that only advanced walkers or race walkers should use the second because you may pick up too much speed and go out of control unless you are an accomplished walker.

Even though I can do both, I prefer the first method and believe you will too. Keep your body erect, almost as if you are leaning backward, away from the slope of the hill. This is a good way to practice erect posture, and it is easy to hold your head up. With your bent arms pumping fast to keep up with your accelerated leg swing, let gravity help pull you down the hill as fast as you can make your legs and feet move in a smooth, coordinated manner. This position also gives you a shorter leg swing, so that your foot doesn't have as far to drop down the hill at heel plant, and this reduces the jarring effect of downhill walking.

The other way to walk downhill is perpendicular to the slope of the hill. The lead leg will get a full swing down the hill for a full stride, and gravity will help you increase momentum. But it is easy for the average exercise walker to pick up too much speed with this method. Unless you can control your posture, technique, and rhythm, you will find you are going downhill fast but sloppily, and maybe out of control.

Question: *When is the best time to walk—morning or evening?*

Answer: The best time is any time you can walk *consistently.* Your body doesn't care whether it is morning, noon, or night. You and your schedule should determine when you walk. Some folks are natural morning people and jump out of bed raring to go. If you are one of these, get up, get a good walk in, shower, have a light, low-fat breakfast, and when you head for work you will be set for a high-energy day.

Conversely, I am a slow starter and would rather ease into the day with breakfast and the newspaper. My preferred time for walking is about an hour before dinner. Walking then reduces your appetite and gives you an exercise-induced caloric afterburn that helps dispose of the evening meal's calories. If you have a stressful job, there isn't any better way than a brisk or aerobic walk to clear your mind and work off frustrations or hostilities that may have accumulated during the day. A vigorous walk after work will energize you physically and soothe you mentally. The often-prescribed chemical tranquilizers cannot do for you what a long, hard walk will do.

Question: *I live in an area where there is a lot of traffic pollution and smog. Are there better times than others to exercise, and how does this affect me?*

Answer: Unfortunately, millions of exercisers live in high-density cities with traffic pollution and/or smog. They should try to walk early in the morning, before the pollution reaches its maximum concentrations.

According to Dr. Bryant Stamford, director of the Health Promotion and Wellness Center and professor of allied health at the School of Medicine, University of Louisville, Kentucky, carbon monoxide and ozone present the biggest threats to exercisers. Exhaust fumes from automobiles are the major contributor to carbon-monoxide pollution. Ozone results from the sun acting on nitrogen dioxide and certain hydrocarbons; it is a predominant component of city smog. In his September 1990 "Exercise Adviser" column for *The Physician and Sportsmedicine*, he stated: "Exercising in heavy traffic places an added strain on the heart, which must work harder to counteract the increased intake of carbon monoxide and decreased oxygen concentration." Dr. Stamford suggested six ways city exercisers can minimize the risks of encountering air pollution:

1. Avoid exercising during peak traffic hours.

2. Avoid exercising when the sun is brightest; ozone levels increase on sunny days.

3. Respect air-pollution alerts and exercise accordingly.

4. Exercise in open areas, where air currents can move about freely, dispersing pollutants.

5. Be aware of exercising or resting for prolonged periods under shade trees; they can trap pollutants.

6. Avoid ambient cigarette smoke before and after exercise. If

you are a smoker, never smoke just after exercise; wait until you are breathing normally. Quitting smoking is even better.

Question: *Is it better to exercise before or after a meal?*

Answer: It is best to exercise before *and* after a meal, but never do intense exercise right after eating. The time for that is an hour or two before, or at least two hours after, eating your meal. I have some of my best and fastest walks when I feel hungry. Vigorous exercise tends to blunt the appetite. When you work up a good sweat in warm weather, you will come in very thirsty but not very hungry. That's when you will drink a lot of fluids (preferably water) and tend to eat less, which helps with weight control.

Exercising vigorously right after a meal is ill-advised. In his "Exercise Adviser" column, Dr. Stamford cautioned: "During vigorous exercise the blood is withdrawn from the abdomen and shunted toward the working muscles. Digestion is put on hold, which can cause considerable distress. . . . Vigorous exercise increases sympathetic nerve stimulation. This speeds the heart rate and increases cardiac output, but it also inhibits movement of the food through the intestines and decreases gastric and pancreatic juice secretions."

Instead of flopping down in front of the TV and letting your eyes glaze over after dinner, take a nice, easy stroll. In the parts of the country that have four distinct seasons, spring, summer, and fall are great strolling months. Dr. Stamford pointed out that slow walking "requires the use of large muscle groups, but doesn't make extreme metabolic demands, so the blood can stay in the abdomen and digestion proceeds. . . . Mild exercise can actually aid the movement of foodstuff through the gastrointestinal tract by speeding the emptying of the stomach and more rapidly relieving that full feeling."

A stroll after dinner has another significant benefit: marital communication. Get away from the TV and telephone. Spend 20 or 30 minutes reestablishing your ability to communicate with each other while strolling along. A walk after dinner is the catalyst for sharing problems and finding solutions. In this hectic world, it might strengthen some frayed marriage bonds.

Question: *Should I breathe in any particular way while walking?*

Answer: Walking at a slow pace doesn't put any demands on breathing except for extremely overweight people. As you pick up your pace, however, particularly if you move on to aerobic walking and race walking, your method of breathing can affect performance. There is a tendency to breathe shallowly, which only supplies air to the upper passages—the mouth, throat, and bronchi. These areas do not participate in the oxygen-gas exchange with the blood. The lungs are where oxygen is transferred to the bloodstream so that it can be pumped out to the muscles by the heart.

As you walk faster and need more oxygen, breathe deeply. Inhale to capacity by *expanding* your stomach as you fill your lungs. Some coaches call this *belly breathing*. Many people try to fill their lungs by sucking in their stomachs as they inhale. To try it both ways, stand up and draw in as much air as possible by expanding your stomach. Let the air out; then draw in as much air as possible by sucking in your stomach. Do you feel the difference? If you fill your lungs several times each way, you'll find that your lungs fill all the way to the top if you expand your stomach. Develop your own comfortable relationship between breathing and stride frequency. Breathe as you need, and breathe deeply. Correct posture with a straight back opens up the rib cage so that your lungs can fill to capacity.

Question: *When I walk real fast, I sometimes get a sharp pain in my side. What is it and what can I do about it?*

Answer: This is the puzzling "side stitch," which seems to defy diagnosis. There are several theories about it, but no clear consensus. The American Running and Fitness Association book *Conquering Athletic Injuries* states: "Because the mechanism of the side-stitch is poorly understood, there is no standard treatment." The baffling thing about side stitches is that they intermittently attack some exercisers but never others.

There are a few consistent clues, however. Side stitches seem to appear more often in exercisers who are building a fitness level than in fully conditioned athletes. They occur near the bottom of the rib cage when the exerciser is at an intense level of exercise, and they usually fade when the intensity drops. I remember getting side stitches off and on when I was building up my fitness. They always went away when I reduced my pace. Side stitches are an uncomfortable annoyance but nothing to worry about. They will probably disappear once you have reached a good fitness level. In the meantime, when one occurs, slow down.

Question: *I sweat a lot when I walk fast in warm weather. How much water should I drink, and do I need any of those special athletic drinks?*

Answer: Unless you are walking for more than an hour or live in a hot climate, the normal recommended intake of six to eight glasses of water a day should be enough. The problem is that very few people—including me—actually drink eight full glasses of water every day. But I know I should, and so should you.

Water makes up about 60 percent of the body weight and is used in a number of body functions, such as digestion, absorption, circulation, excretion, nutrient transmission, tissue maintenance, and temperature regulation. Besides sweat, you lose water from the body in urine, feces, and when you exhale. Drinking lots of water year round, not merely when you sweat, is a healthful thing to do.

Some of your daily water requirements can come from juices, fruits, and vegetables that have a high water content, as well as caffeine-free soft drinks. Coffee and tea (decaffeinated or regular), caffeinated soft drinks, and alcohol do not count as water intake. Alcohol causes dehydration, and the other drinks are diuretics that actually make you lose fluid. Some herbal teas may also be diuretics.

Sports drinks like Gatorade, which you see along the sidelines at football games and sporting events, are expensive relative to water and unnecessary for the average exerciser. They are some-times called electrolyte-replacement drinks because they contain sodium and potassium, which help balance the acidity-alkalinity of fluids in the body cells. But the *University of California at Berkeley Wellness Letter* pointed out that "most sports drinks ac-tually contain far less potassium than a glass of orange juice." It added: "There is rarely any need to replace electrolytes by con-suming special 'sport drinks' or mineral supplements. These min-erals are lost in small quantities that can easily be replaced by a normal diet." Further, "The sugar content in most of these drinks is excessive." All things considered, it's hard to beat plain water.

There are a lot of bottled waters on the market, and some of them are not as safe as or any better than the tap water from a well-regulated municipal source. In some cities, however, the water may taste a little odd, so people buy bottled water. The *University of California at Berkeley Wellness Letter* recommended refrigerating tap water in a closed container to enhance its flavor. Also, "A simple aerator at the end of your faucet can improve flat-tasting water."

At times I want to drink something fizzy, and plain water doesn't fill the bill. I keep a couple of bottles of plain seltzer water in the refrigerator. This is nothing more than purified, carbonated water. It has no sodium added, like club soda, which may contain 30 to 65 milligrams per 8 ounces. You can squeeze some lime or lemon in plain seltzer. I sometimes put about a third of a glass of orange juice in it for my own inexpensive, healthful homemade "sport drink."

Question: *How much should I warm up and cool down?*

Answer: A low-intensity stroll at a 20-minute-mile pace or slower doesn't require any warm-up. Simply start walking, find your comfort zone, and continue. The moderate-intensity brisk walker will probably find that a 17- to 19-minute-mile pace feels best for the first ¼ to ½ mile before moving into the full brisk pace. The high-intensity aerobic walker will be more fit and can easily handle a 14-minute-mile pace from the start for a warm-up pace, gradually increasing speed after the first ½ mile.

Fast walkers generally agree that their first mile is their most sluggish. It takes almost a mile before the leg muscles really get warmed up, loose, and rhythmic. After a mile, aerobic walkers, and even brisk walkers, will find another level of speed that seems more effortless. On my 5-mile walks, my third, fourth, and fifth miles are the smoothest and fastest, and they seem to require less effort than the first. If you start at a faster pace than I have suggested, you won't injure yourself, but you probably will find that the first mile requires more effort than the rest of your walk.

The cool down for a walker is less of a problem than for a runner. Strollers don't really have any cooling down to do, but they should stretch at the end of their walk—as should all walkers. On a hot day brisk walkers may want to stroll for a couple of hundred yards to cool down. Aerobic walkers should drop their arms from the bent-arm swing and stroll for 5 or 10 minutes to let their heart rates drop. If for any reason your heart rate doesn't return to normal in about 10 minutes, it would be wise to consult your physician.

FIGURE 11.2A   **FIGURE 11.2B**

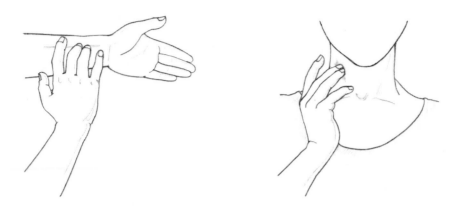

Question: *What is the best way to check my pulse so I will know if I am in my aerobic-training range? How often should I check it?*

Answer: It is difficult to get an accurate heart rate when exercising, and if you stop, your heart rate drops quickly (or it should), which also contributes to inaccuracy. I find that it is nearly impossible to get a good reading wearing a wristwatch with a sweep-second hand. I suggest you invest in a cheap digital watch, which will help you not only check your pulse but time your walk down to the second (which is helpful if you are going a measured distance and trying to improve your time). Most discount stores have digital watches with all the features you need for $20 or less.

Checking your pulse can be done either at your wrist (on the thumb side, see Figure 11.2A), or at the large artery (the carotid artery) that runs up either side of your neck just below and a bit in front of the back corner of your jaw (see Figure 11.2B). While you are reading this, familiarize yourself with these two points. Place the middle fingers of your opposite hand between the wristbone and the ligaments in the center of your arm on the thumb side of your wrist. You should be able to feel your pulse beating. Also probe lightly on your neck to feel your pulse in that artery.

I found that the neck artery was the best for me when I started walking and checked my pulse every day, but people with considerable fat around the neck may have trouble finding their pulse there. The easiest way to check your heart rate is to take your pulse for 10 seconds, then multiply by 6. You can also take your pulse for 15 seconds and multiply by 4.

If you are a beginner and want to walk with your heart in your aerobic-training range, I suggest you take your pulse after 10 minutes into your walk. Do it while walking; don't stop. Your heart rate should be within your aerobic-training range after 10 minutes if you are walking fast enough. Don't be surprised if it isn't. Walking is deceptive, and often you think you are working harder than your heart rate indicates. The one major exception to this is obese walkers, whose heart rates will rise quickly at a modest pace.

As you approach the end of your walk, but before you stop, quickly take your pulse again. If it is still in the aerobic-training range and if you maintained your pace steadily enough to keep it in that range for at least 20 minutes, you have gotten an aerobic workout.

How often you should check your pulse depends on your exercise goals. If you are seeking only a modest fitness level, you needn't check it at all. Simply walk at a comfortable pace for the distance in miles, or for the duration in minutes, that you want. However, if you intend to reach the aerobic fitness of a jogger by exercise walking or want to burn as many calories per minute as possible, it is important to know that your heart rate is in your aerobic-training range. In such instances, I suggest that in the beginning you take your pulse every time you walk to familiarize yourself with your walking pace as it relates to your heart rate. Once you get beyond the 15-minute-mile brisk pace, a strong, consistent walking speed is required to be aerobic. Your heart will let you know if you are walking too fast or too slowly. The chances are that it will be the latter.

I mentioned that I *used* to take my heart rate. By this I mean I have become so familiar with my pace, heart rate, and fitness level over the past few years (and about 10,000 miles) that I can now walk my 5-mile hilly course and know within about 5 beats where my heart rate is without actually checking it. Once you achieve a high level of fitness, you can do the same if you took your heart rate regularly in the beginning and matched it to your pace. It is important to get to know your heart rate and all your body's signals.

Once in a while someone downplays the importance of heart

rate when exercising. But if your heart has to work hard for you to do very little exercise, it is telling you that you are not in good shape. Wouldn't you want to know that?

Question: *I've read about heart-rate monitors. Are they any good, and how much do they cost?*

Answer: There are several kinds of heart-rate monitors: the kind that clips onto your ear, the kind that has a small cuff that fits over your finger, and the more expensive wireless unit with electrodes attached to a chest band which transmits your pulse signal to a receiver in a unit that you wear on your wrist. This unit is about like an oversized digital watch.

The finger and ear units are much cheaper but have a number of drawbacks, one of which is accuracy. If you aren't going to be totally accurate, you can get close enough by taking your pulse the way I just described. You might as well put your money into another pair of walking shoes. If you are going to become a serious aerobic walker, however, or if you have a major weight problem and realize you are going to have to do a lot of walking to get the pounds off and keep them off, a wireless heart-rate monitor is a good investment. And I do mean investment; at 1991 prices it will cost in the neighborhood of $200.

My first exposure to monitors was at the Cooper Wellness Program. There the staff put them on all overweight participants or on those who had some heart-related abnormality. The purpose was to make sure that the exerciser was not doing too much too soon.

Ava Bursau, director of the Wellness Program, has tested a number of the wireless units and for the past several years has used the Computer Instruments Corporation (CIC) Pro-Trainer model. She finds it is easy for people to learn how to use, and the big numbers are easy for older participants to read. She also likes it because it is accurate. Some participants could be in a life-threatening situation if they put too much stress on their heart, so accuracy is critical.

The CIC Pro-Trainer has a dual-display digital receiver, which shows the pulse either at a given moment or over elapsed time. Its memory records the amount of time spent below, in, and above the programmed target zone. It also has high- and low-limit alarms. This last feature is important for an obese walker.

Heart-rate monitors can be a safeguard for extremely overweight people who are starting a walking program. I remember Jerry from New York City in a class I had at the Wellness Program in 1990. He was 41 years old, 5 feet, 10 inches, 293 pounds, with 36 percent body fat. He tested poorly on his stress test, had extremely high blood pressure, and was a smoker. He also had a passion for corned beef, pastrami, and chocolate cheesecake. If he didn't change his life-style, it was unlikely that he would see many more birthdays. He knew this and was trying hard to get his life on a healthy path.

I asked Jerry to walk several laps on the indoor track at the Aerobics Center to check his posture, technique, and rhythm. For his size he moved extremely well; we were going so slowly, however, that I was walking sideways and sometimes even backward as I observed and coached him. Even though we were walking considerably less than a 20-minute-mile pace, he was breathing heavily, and his heart-rate monitor alarm went off at 152 beats per minute, which was 85 percent of his aerobic-training range.

I had my heart-rate monitor on that day, as I do from time to time to compare my pulse with various class participants' at different fitness levels and walking paces. I glanced at my wrist unit; my pulse was only 93. Even though I was 21 years older than Jerry, my fitness level was 59 heartbeats less at our walking pace. The heart-rate-monitor alarm was a safety signal for Jerry to slow his pace down even more. In time, as the pounds come off, Jerry will be able to pick up his walking speed, but he was not yet ready to walk faster.

For a moderate-intensity walker, a heart-rate monitor may not be worth the money, but for someone who wants to be an aggressive aerobic walker, it probably is. For anyone who is walking for weight control, particularly someone who is obese and wants to be safe and yet walk at the upper end of his training range, a monitor is worth having. Creative Health Products, Inc. (1-800-742-4478) will send you a catalog listing the heart-rate monitors it sells.

Question: *What do you think of pedometers?*
Answer: My experience with pedometers has not been good. Over the past five years, three have been given to me as gifts. When I checked them against an accurate measured mile, they registered a longer distance by as much as ²⁄₁₀ of a mile. In a 3-mile walk, this would be an error of more than ½ mile. A car odometer will

give you a more accurate distance measurement, and all you have to remember are your key ½-mile points.

I am a stickler for distance accuracy, because I time a lot of my walks, so I bought a Measure Master wheel made by the Rolatape Corporation of Spokane, Washington. Various handyman catalogs carry them for about $89 (1991 price). They are accurate down to ¹⁄₁₀ of a foot. I have my 5-mile country course marked every ¼ mile by a small spray-painted Day-Glo orange dot near the bottom of a fence post or tree, or at the side of the road.

If you have a walking club or a neighborhood group that walks a set course, or even several courses, it is better for the group to buy one of these measuring wheels than for several people to buy pedometers, which would probably cost more.

Question: *What about walking to music—does it help?*

Answer: I think walking to music helps in every way, and next to a good pair of walking shoes I believe a Sony Walkman is the best long-term investment an exercise walker can make. I have referred often to the *rhythm* of walking, and nothing helps this better than music. Many women tell me that walking to music makes them walk not only more but also faster.

Walkers moving beyond the brisk pace to the 12-minute-mile aerobic pace will definitely become looser and more fluid if they have a good music beat to drive them. Music reduces the mechanical action of the walking gait by increasing the rhythmic flow of the walker. Even slower walkers find their exercise time passes more quickly with the soothing, entertaining beat of their favorite music.

I grew up with the big-band sounds of Glenn Miller, Tommy Dorsey, and Harry James, and on my walks I often get lost in the nostalgia of my youth. These are some of my best walks. Each generation has its music and the special memories associated with it. Take your music with you on your walk, and you will move more smoothly, faster, and more happily than you ever thought possible.

If you invest in a Walkman, I suggest you get one with an AM/FM radio, along with the auto-reverse feature for the cassette. When traveling, you may not want to take your cassettes along, so the radio lets you pick up local stations. The auto-reverse feature plays a whole tape without your having to slow down to turn it over. It is also worth a few dollars extra to buy rechargeable batteries and a recharger. If you do much walking, over time they will save you money.

My most important advice to anyone who uses a Walkman is *never, ever carry it in your hand*. This is a major mistake made by many people. Although the Walkman is light, subconsciously it will cause you to alter your arm swing. In the spring of 1990, at a walking clinic in a big shopping mall in Dallas, I was checking the technique of a young woman who had just purchased a pair of new walking shoes, and I said that she must be left-handed. She was a fast walker who used the bent-arm swing, but her right arm did not swing with the same vigor as her left. When she told me she was right-handed, I was stunned. Then she told me that the only thing she was doing differently was that she didn't have her Walkman with her, which she takes on all her walks and carries in her right hand. This is a perfect example of how hand-carrying a Walkman altered a dominant arm swing so much that the dominant arm had less vigor than the subdominant arm.

A properly balanced arm swing is essential for all walkers, but especially for brisk and aerobic walkers. If you are going to use a Walkman, carry it in a small fanny pack so that your hands are unencumbered and your arms get a complete swing cycle. Carol has a fanny pack, but I use an old belt and leave the Walkman hooked onto it. I can strap the belt over my sweats or shorts and be ready to go. However, a fanny pack keeps your Walkman from getting wet if you're caught in the rain, and it carries extra cassettes.

When wearing a Walkman, be aware that you may not be able to hear cars coming from behind. You can also become absorbed in your music and not check carefully for oncoming vehicles at an intersection. Do not become musically preoccupied and forget about traffic safety.

12 WEIGHT CONTROL WITH WALKING

I suspect that at least 60 percent of the people reading this book are involved in either a weight-loss effort or a weight-maintenance program. I am one of the latter. I have gained and lost several hundred pounds over the past thirty years, and, as mentioned in Chapter 1, at one time was 52 pounds heavier and four suit sizes larger than I am today. At age 64 I weigh 182 pounds, exactly what I weighed at age 22.

Since I have put together the right combination of exercise walking and diet, my weight hasn't fluctuated 2 pounds over eight years. I have won my battle . . . finally. The successful solution to my weight problem, yours, and everybody else's boils down to two factors: (1) diet composition (low-fat, high-complex carbohydrates); (2) exercise (the right kind with adequate frequency, duration, and intensity). It is a dead heat as to which is more important, but it is a matter of record that those who have managed their weight problems the longest invariably are exercisers. The importance of diet will be discussed in the next chapter, but first let's tackle the one that is more difficult for everyone: exercise.

In a January 1991 *People* magazine article about Oprah Winfrey regaining the 67 pounds she lost on her highly publicized liquid diet, Dr. Keith Berndtson, a weight-management specialist at Rush-Presbyterian–St. Luke's Medical Center in Chicago, stated: "The rate of regain on any weight loss regimen—not just liquid food replacement—is a whopping 95 percent, unless paired with exercise." According to *People*, Oprah had stopped exercising regularly and had gone back to eating her favorite foods, which are high in fat.

Most experts agree that exercise is essential for successful weight loss. In an April 30, 1990, *Newsweek* story on the liquid diet fad, Dr. Peter Wood of Stanford's Center for Research in Disease Prevention said: "A diet program that does not incorporate physical activity is probably doomed to failure." Oprah made a comment in *People* that goes to the heart of the problem: "I didn't do whatever the maintenance program was. I thought I was cured." Unfortunately, there is no cure for a weight, cholesterol, or alcohol problem. The problem always remains; one can only work to control it, and such control must be maintained one day at a time for the rest of your life.

Yesterday's control was a victory, today's control is a battle being fought, and tomorrow's control is a new battle facing you. The role of exercise in these battles cannot be overstated. Consistent exercisers, particularly exercise walkers, develop resolve, discipline, and an uncommon ability to take command of their lifestyle and make the changes necessary to control their problem. Oprah didn't have a chance to succeed without exercise, and neither do you.

"When you examine long-time weight losers versus those who gain their weight back, the difference is always exercise," said Charles P. Lucas, clinical professor of medicine at Wayne State University School of Medicine in Detroit in *The Physician and Sportsmedicine* magazine. Dr. Lucas, who is also chief of the Division of Preventive and Nutritional Medicine at William Beaumont Hospital in Royal Oak, Michigan, added, "Long-term weight losers are still exercising on average 3.3 hours a week after several years." People exercise for various reasons, and the amount of exercise that might be beneficial for one part of the body may not be sufficient for consistent weight loss or weight maintenance. Dr. Lucas pointed out that exercising three times a week is good for cardiovascular fitness, but "for metabolic fitness and weight control it is necessary to exercise nearly every day."

The reason exercise is more difficult to sustain than dieting is that it takes time, effort, and consistency. Dieting, on the other hand, is passive, and, while it requires enormous mental discipline, it does not require exertion or the interruption of daily activities. For instance, you can be dieting while reading this book or watching a movie, but you couldn't be exercising.

UNDERSTANDING FAT

There is no need to rush headlong into an exercise or diet program in an effort to lose fat unless you first understand its role in your physiological makeup. You don't cure excess fat, you control it, and what works sensationally for one person may be only moderately successful for another. In most cases the threshold of expectation about getting rid of excess fat exceeds the realities of how it can be done. Impatience is the biggest enemy of those in a weight-loss program. Most don't really understand how their weight is accumulated and stored or how it must be broken down chemically and used by the body as fuel to be eliminated.

Fat plays an important role in how our bodies function; it is only *excess* fat that creates problems. The textbook *Exercise Physiology* points out that the most noteworthy functions of body fat include (1) providing the body's largest store of potential energy; (2) serving as a cushion for the protection of vital organs; (3) providing insulation from the thermal stress of cold. For all intents and purposes, it is number 1 that raises havoc. Most overweight people are simply storing more energy every day than they are using. The exceptions, of course, are those who have a glandular or other specific medical reason for their excess weight, but they represent a very small percentage of the population.

Apples and Pears

If you are carrying excess body fat, are you shaped like an apple or a pear? The difference may determine your health risk and may influence your success in getting rid of fat by dieting and exercise. In the January 1991 issue of *The Physician and Sportsmedicine*, Dr. Bryant Stamford discussed in detail the apple- and pear-shape fat accumulation: "Obese men tend to be shaped like apples, storing their fat above the waist, in the nape of the neck, shoulders, and abdomen. . . . Obese women on the other hand tend to be shaped like pears, storing their fat lower on the body, on the buttocks, and thighs." This arrangement is also interchangeable, according to Stamford; men can be shaped like pears and women like apples.

The apples have good news and bad news. The good news is that they are able to reduce fat more easily than pears. The bad news is that the apple's fat poses increased heart-attack risks and the propensity to develop diabetes. The excess dietary fat that is stored by apples is controlled by active enzymes. (The dictionary defines *enzymes* as "any of various proteins, as pepsin, originating from living cells and capable of producing certain chemical changes in organic substances by catalytic action, as in digestion.") According to Dr. Stamford, enzyme activity plays a role in calling fat from storage to be used as fuel.

Dr. Stamford stated: "Active enzymes may contribute to high cholesterol levels in apples because the greater amount of fat stored in the gut, the greater amount that can be dumped into the blood stream. . . . Enzyme activity increases when adrenalin is released during times of emotional stress and exercise stress causes fat stored in the abdominal cavity to be released into the blood stream."

This process creates a mixed blessing. Exercising is good because it shunts blood flow toward the working muscles, fueling them with the fat you want to shed. But, as Dr. Stamford pointed out, during emotional stress this is bad, because fat-laden blood from the apple area is routed directly to the liver, providing it with abundant raw material for the production of artery-clogging cholesterol.

Additional bad news for apples is that abdominal fat cells tend to be larger than those in other areas of the body. Large fat cells are associated with glucose intolerance and an excess of insulin in the blood, which can develop into diabetes. In addition, "Excess insulin may promote reabsorption of sodium by the kidney, which may in turn lead to high blood pressure."

Metabolic problems such as high cholesterol and glucose intolerance increase the risk of coronary heart disease for apples. But nature seems to provide an escape hatch for some of the bad-news scenarios. Because the abdominal fat cells are so active and the turnover rate for abdominal fat is high, apples are able to reduce their abdominal fat more easily than pears are able to reduce fat on their hips, thighs, and buttocks.

There's more good news for apples. A study has shown that when fat is lost as a result of exercise, more is lost from the trunk area, where apples carry their weight, than from the extremities. Dr. Stamford said: "The message for apples is clear: Get moving!" I'll add: You can walk that gut off in less time than you think. You will not only look and feel better but also reduce your risk of heart attack, diabetes, and high blood pressure.

While pears don't face the health risks that apples do, the fat they are carrying is more stubborn and harder to lose. Dr. Stamford referred to this fat as "gluteal-femoral pattern obesity." Over and over in my walking clinics women ask, "Is walking good for reducing my hips and thighs?" All women seem to be preoccupied with the size of their hips and thighs, but no exercise will spot-reduce a particular area of the body. The best any exercise can do is to help burn the body's excess fat, including that from hips and thighs. In this regard, exercise walking is the best exercise of all.

Research suggests that the reason fat is so stubborn on females is that the gluteal-femoral cells cling to their fat except during lactation. Dr. Stamford said: "This suggests that the female body zealously guards fat stores to ensure adequate energy support for nursing a baby." Further studies have found that exercise training without calorie restriction reduces body fat in men but not in women.

It seems that the deck is stacked against women who want to maintain their girlish figures. Childbirth brings on the most stubborn fat and puts it in the most obvious places, but nature gives women the escape hatch just mentioned. Over and over I have said that women are natural walkers, much better than men. The combination of a low-fat diet (see next chapter) and exercise walking will ultimately take fat off hips, thighs, and everywhere else. I guarantee it!

UNLOADING EXCESS-FAT FUEL

Filling the fat cells with more fuel than the body needs is generally a process of long-term, pleasurable overindulgence. Cheeseburgers, french fries, malted milk shakes, pizzas, cheesecake, and other heavy-fat foods did their job, and we loved every minute of it. Breaking all the excess fat down biochemically so that the body can use it as fuel is time-consuming and not always enjoyable or swift. Even if you are successful in getting it done by self-denial or some bizarre diet program, there is the specter of the 95 percent failure rate for keeping excess fat out of those cells for the rest of your life.

Exercise and altered diet composition, plus modest calorie restriction, are the surest ways to burn the excess fat that has accumulated in your cells. It is a slow process, but to be effective in the long term it *should* be. Stop for a moment and estimate how long it took you to put all that excess fuel into your fat cells. Was it 5, 10, or 20 years? In the lectures I conduct at the Cooper Wellness Program, I ask this question. The average age of the participants is 48, and it is a rarity that anyone in the group has put on all of his or her excess weight in 5 years or less; usually it has taken at least 10 years.

The 1985 guidelines for appropriate weight loss were 1 to 2 pounds per week. The *Tufts University Diet and Nutrition Letter* reported in its January 1991 issue that ½ to 1 pound per week is the new guideline: "The slower the weight is taken off, the more likely it will be to stay off." There are two factors at work in this sentence. First, you should not jolt your metabolic system with extreme calorie restrictions. Losing slowly is the healthy way. Second, and equally important, a permanent weight loss must be accompanied by a changed life-style that includes reduced fat intake and regular exercise. Life-styles are not changed quickly. If you have the patience and determination to lose weight slowly while adapting to a new life-style, by the time you reach your weight goal, everything will be in place for it to become your permanent weight.

There are also new recommended adult weight ranges, which are somewhat higher than before. Maybe you have a weight problem; maybe you don't. Table 12.1 shows the new guidelines issued in 1990 by the U.S. Departments of Agriculture and Health and Human Services. These guidelines are meant to take the focus off appearance and to emphasize the health problems associated with too much or too little weight. From a health standpoint, a slightly higher weight range is acceptable for adults 35 years of age and older than was previously recommended.

Dr. C. Wayne Callaway, a member of the committee that developed the new guidelines and clinical professor of medicine at George Washington University, said, "We don't want consumers to just look at the chart. . . . Our definition of healthy weight says you also have to know your other health numbers, such as blood cholesterol and blood pressure and then consider them along with

TABLE 12.1.

Suggested weights for adults

HEIGHT*	WEIGHT IN POUNDS†	
	19 to 34 years	*35 years and older*
5'0"	97–128	108–138
5'1"	101–132	111–143
5'2"	104–137	115–148
5'3"	107–141	119–152
5'4"	111–146	122–157
5'5"	114–150	126–162
5'6"	118–155	130–167
5'7"	121–160	134–172
5'8"	125–164	138–178
5'9"	129–169	142–183
5'10"	132–174	146–188
5'11"	136–179	151–194
6'0"	140–184	155–199
6'1"	144–189	159–205
6'2"	148–195	164–210
6'3"	152–200	168–216
6'4"	156–205	173–222
6'5"	160–211	177–228

* Without shoes
† Without clothes
SOURCE: U.S. Department of Agriculture, U.S. Department of Health and Human Services

weight." Dr. Callaway was saying that if you are a little overweight according to the weight chart, but all your other numbers are on target, the extra pounds may be less of an issue than they would be if your cholesterol and blood pressure were also high. Remember too that where the weight is being carried is important. Apples have more to worry about than pears.

One pound of body fat equals 3,500 calories. This means that, if you are 25 pounds overweight, through the combination of exercise and calorie restriction you have to somehow create a deficit of 87,500 calories ($25 \times 3,500 = 87,500$). This number may seem enormous and unattainable, but think how many people try to do it by diet alone. That is *really* doing it the hard way.

Creating a calorie shortfall of 87,500 by exercise and slow-weight-loss dieting becomes a very doable daily project. The latter will be discussed in detail in the next chapter, but a realistic goal should be to split the expected shortfall equally between calorie reduction (diet) and extra calorie expenditure (exercise). Thus, in an effort to lose the 25 pounds or 87,500 calories at a rate of approximately 1 pound (3,500 calories) a week, you only need to reduce your calorie intake by 250 calories a day. This reduction totals 1,750 calories (7 × 250 = 1,750) a week, which is one half of your weekly goal. You now need to exercise away 1,750 calories for your weekly calorie shortfall of 3,500 or about 1 pound of weight loss.

This neat mathematical equation of weight loss will not occur with exact precision for everyone; it is only a realistic approximation. You might be pleasantly surprised to find that you lose more than a pound a week if you are an apple, or may be disappointed when you lose less if you have the stubborn fat of a pear. Don't be in a hurry, however, and raise your expectations too high. Even if it takes 30 weeks instead of 25 to reach your goal, that is only about seven months. I'll bet you didn't put on those 25 pounds in seven months, so why expect to take them off any sooner?

For many people, a lifetime exercise program is a major stumbling block. "I don't have the time" is the excuse used most frequently. In a country where the average family spends about seven hours a day watching television, this has a hollow ring to it. In fact, for the blue-collar group, who are the most overweight and underexercised of all, it is a tragically weak excuse. They watch more TV than anyone.

Spinning off 1,750 calories per week is going to take about 4 hours. There are 168 hours in each week. Anyone truly interested in long-term weight loss must find 48 minutes for five out of seven days to exercise. Actually, half of the 4 hours can be done in two days (Saturday and Sunday) for an hour a day, which means that the rest could be done in four days at only 30 minutes a day.

I have found that busy, motivated people who are truly committed to permanent weight loss and a permanent life-style change almost without exception find a way to get in their necessary amount of exercise. Conversely, those with more time but who are not deeply motivated or convinced that exercise is part of the solution will always cite a lack of time. There are also a great number of nonexercisers who use this excuse because they don't like any of the recommended exercises. The quick burnouts from exercise machines and those injured by jogging fall into this category.

In reality none of us is going to do something that we don't like for very long, particularly a voluntary make-work activity like exercise. For this reason, exercise walking has the greatest adherence and lowest dropout rates. Being natural, injury free, and enjoyable makes it the exercise of choice for anyone attempting to lose weight and keep it off permanently. Regular exercise must become part of a changed life-style. Dieting by itself simply won't burn all your excess fat on a permanent basis.

Evidence of the limited possibilities of extensive calorie restriction is cited in *Exercise Physiology*: "In the United States, the caloric intake per person has steadily decreased over the past 80 years, yet body weight and body fat have slowly increased. . . . Americans now eat 5–10% fewer calories than they did 15 years ago, yet they weigh an average of 5 pounds more." Certainly if dieting were effective, this reduction in caloric intake should bring the national body weight to a lower level.

Over the past 80 years, however, at home and at work we have been chipping away at the amount of physical activity required to function. By various household and workplace inventions, plus alternative locomotion systems, we have found more and more ways to substitute natural gas, electricity, and petroleum energy for our own. We have tilted the delicate balance between energy expenditure and food intake in the wrong direction. To get that balance back requires exercise, and exercise walking is all that's needed.

Exercise Physiology states: "Evidence is accumulating to support the contention that exercise may be more effective than dieting for long-term weight control." The textbook indicates that it is becoming increasingly clear that people who maintain a physically active life-style or who become involved in endurance exercise programs maintain a desirable level of body composition. "Within this framework, a strong case can be made for habitual, vigorous physical activity for individuals of all ages."

LOSING FAT, GAINING MUSCLE, AND BURNING CALORIES

The use of exercise in a weight-loss program has a two-pronged favorable effect. In addition to burning excess fat, exercise helps the body develop lean muscle tissue. It helps you alter your body's composition away from a high percentage of fat, which encourages more fat storage, to a leaner, higher ratio of muscle to body weight. And muscle tissue burns more calories than fat does. Your weight-loss objective should not be just to lose weight but to lose fat and gain muscle.

Exercise Physiology says: "When considering exercise for weight control, factors such as frequency, intensity, and duration as well as the specific form of exercise, must be considered." It points out that continuous, big-muscle, aerobic activities that have a moderate to high caloric cost are the best. According to the textbook, "total energy expended" is the most important factor in the effectiveness of an exercise program for weight control.

The energy cost of a weight-bearing exercise such as walking is proportional to body weight. For instance, a 225-pound person will burn more calories than a 150-pound person when both are walking at the same pace.

The importance of burning 300 calories per exercise session is stressed in *Exercise Physiology*: "Although it is difficult to speculate precisely, as to a threshold energy expenditure for weight reduction and fat, *it is generally recommended that the calorie burning effect of each exercise session should be at least 300 calories* [emphasis in original]. . . . This can be achieved with 20 to 30 minutes of moderate-to-vigorous running, swimming, or bicycling or walking for 40 to 60 minutes." Exercise programs of lower caloric cost usually show little or no effect on body weight or body composition.

As has been pointed out repeatedly, the exercise community continually downgrades walking as a vigorous or intensive exercise. *Exercise Physiology* has just done it again by saying that you can burn 300 calories in 20 to 30 minutes with moderate to vigorous running, swimming, or bicycling, but that it takes 40 to 60 minutes to do the same with walking. Two important criteria have been omitted in this comment: (1) the intensity of the walker; (2) the weight of the walker. Both of these affect caloric expenditure.

FIGURE 12.1

Energy expenditure walking on the level at different speeds. Different symbols represent the mean values from various studies reported in the literature

WALKING

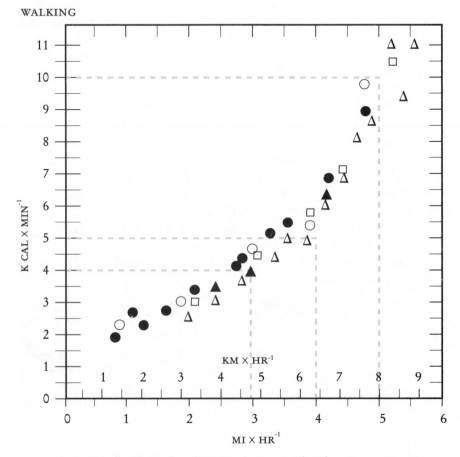

SOURCE: W.D. McArdle, F.I. Katch, and V.L. Katch, *Exercise Physiology: Energy, Nutrition, and Human Performance.* Philadelphia: Lee & Febiger, 1986.

Figure 12.1 displays research results from five countries on the energy expenditure of men who walked at speeds ranging from less than 1.0 mile per hour (slower than 60 minutes per mile) to 6.2 miles per hour (faster than a 10-minute mile). The different symbols in the chart represent the averages from the various studies, and I added the dotted lines to make it easy for you to see where calories burned per minute intersects with the speed of the walkers. This intersection is extremely important because it clearly shows that walking intensity affects calories burned per minute of walking. Beyond the brisk pace of 15-minute miles (4 miles per hour), walking intensity has a dramatic effect. Between a 20-minute mile (3 miles per hour) and a 15-minute mile, there is only a 1-calorie-per-minute difference in energy expenditure. However, increasing the walker's speed just 1 more mile per hour (the aerobic high-intensity pace of 12-minute miles) almost doubled the calories burned per minute in this study.

Exercise Physiology states: "At faster speeds walking becomes less efficient and the relationship curves in an upward direction that indicates a greater caloric cost per unit of distance traveled." You bet it does! Once you move beyond the brisk 15-minute mile, you are in "extended gait" territory, the area where gait *inefficiency* takes over. The walking gait becomes highly inefficient, but, if you shift to running instead of walking faster, you change to a more efficient, calorie-saving gait. The increased walking intensity in Figure 12.1 of only 1 mile per hour from 4 to 5 miles per hour shows what a dramatic increase in calories burned per minute can occur when walking intensity is increased to the aerobic range.

Getting this message across, however, is not easy. The exercise-walking movement finally grew enough in the late 1980s for *The Walking Magazine* to be launched. The January–February 1990 issue had an article about a study conducted at the University of Massachusetts Medical Center in which 80 men and women combined a low-fat diet with a prescribed walking regimen. As you might expect, the results were excellent, but a box in the article answered the question "How fast should you walk?" It said: "The number of calories you burn depends more on how *far* you walk rather than the *speed* at which you walk." This answer is easily disproved by using the graph in Figure 12.1.

Assume that three people of equal weight walked a distance of 10 miles. As in Figure 12.1, their speeds varied: one person walked at 3 miles per hour, another at 4, and the third at 5. Which one burned the most calories? Obviously the fastest walker burned the most calories by a substantial margin, and did it in considerably less time. So you see that with walking you can reduce your exercise time for energy expenditure by increasing your walking speed.

The actual numbers on the extra caloric expenditure and exercise time saved by the fastest walker are impressive. The 20-minute-mile (3-miles-per-hour) walker walked for 200 minutes (10 miles × 20 = 200). At 4 calories burned per minute, this walker burned 800 calories. The 15-minute mile (4-miles-per-hour) walker walked 150 minutes (10 miles × 15 = 150). At 5 calories burned per minute, he burned 750 calories—almost the same number of calories as the 20-minute-mile walker—but in 50 minutes less time. This is a reduction of almost an hour by simply walking at the very doable brisk pace instead of strolling.

Walking the aerobic 12-minute mile (5 miles per hour) pays off handsomely in both extra caloric expenditure *and* exercise time saved. This walker walked the 10 miles in 120 minutes (10 miles × 12 = 120). At 10 calories burned per minute, he burned 1,200 calories, 400 calories *more* than the 20-minute-mile walker and in a whopping 1 hour and 20 minutes less exercise time. Even against the 15-minute-mile walker, he burned 450 more calories in a half hour less. A very productive half hour!

The study in Figure 12.1 used male walkers, but the study at the Institute for Aerobics Research was the first large study using women at walking speeds all the way up to 12-minute miles. I reported the percentages of their caloric expenditure based on walking speed in Chapter 4. In Figure 12.2, you can see how the results look on a chart prepared by Dr. John Duncan. Proving that gait efficiency is not gender-related, these women's caloric expenditures mirrored those of the men in Figure 12.1. The calorie-expenditure-per-minute scale shows that the aerobic 12-minute milers burned more than twice as many calories per minute walking as the 20-minute-mile strollers did.

In sum, walking speed is unquestionably related to energy expenditure for both males and females.

I stipulated in the caloric computation of the theoretical 10-mile walkers used with Figure 12.1 that they be of equal weight. Table 12.2 computed energy expenditure based on speed of walking (on a level surface) and body weight. It indicates that there is also a definite relationship between walking speed, body weight, and energy expenditure.

As stated in *Exercise Physiology*, these figures are accurate within 15 percent for both men and women of different sizes. The textbook suggests that the error rate would be only about 50 to 100 calories for someone walking 2 hours each day. For heavier individuals, extrapolations can be made, albeit with some loss in

FIGURE 12.2

Walking for fitness—walking for health: How much is enough?

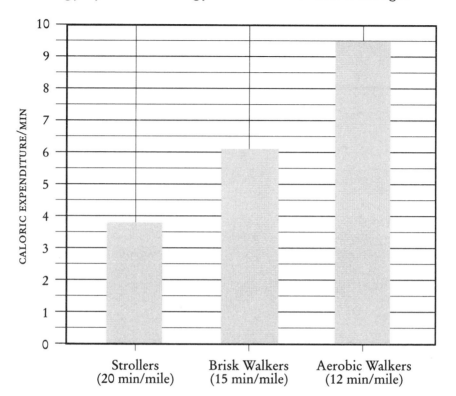

SOURCE: NaturalSport Walking Study, Institue for Aerobics Research, Dallas, Texas.

accuracy. You may wish to figure your own calorie expenditure per minute by checking the boldface miles-per-hour column against the boldface pounds column. For instance, if you are 180 pounds and walk at 3 miles per hour, you could expect to burn about 4.8 calories per minute.

This table is fine as far as it goes; unfortunately, it does not go far enough in terms of walking speed since it stops at 4 miles per hour. The most impressive numbers for calories burned per minute of walking occur at 5 miles per hour, as shown in Figures 12.1 and 12.2. This is one more indication that the exercise community

TABLE 12.2.

Prediction of energy expenditure (kcal · min⁻¹) based on speed of walking and body weight*

SPEED			BODY WEIGHT						
mph	km · hr⁻¹	kg	36	45	54	64	73	82	91
		lbs	80	100	120	140	160	180	200
2.0	3.22		1.9	2.2	2.6	2.9	3.2	3.5	3.8
2.5	4.02		2.3	2.7	3.1	3.5	3.8	4.2	4.5
3.0	4.83		2.7	3.1	3.6	4.0	4.4	4.8	5.3
3.5	5.63		3.1	3.6	4.2	4.6	5.0	5.4	6.1
4.0	6.44		3.5	4.1	4.7	5.2	5.8	6.4	7.0

* Data from R. Passmore and J. V. G. A. Durnin, "Human Energy Expenditure." *Physiol. Rev.* 35:801, 1955.
SOURCE: W. D. McArdle, F. I. Katch, and V. L. Katch, *Exercise Physiology: Energy, Nutrition, and Human Performance.* Philadelphia: Lea & Febiger, 1986.

believes people can't or won't walk faster than a 15-minute mile. At that point we are advised to run, cycle, swim, or do some other "vigorous" exercise—instead of simply walking faster.

The same speed and duration may not be as effective when you near your weight-loss goal as it was when you started. For example, if you are trying to lose 40 pounds, you will probably have to increase your walking duration and/or speed after you have lost 10 or 15 pounds in order to maintain the same rate of calorie burn per minute. That is a happy dilemma, however, if you are getting close to your goal weight. In a big weight-loss program, the last 10 pounds are always the toughest and seem to take forever. Perhaps at this point you will want to really turn on the walking speed and increase your calories burned per minute. By then you will be lighter and more physically fit, so go for it!

Exercise professionals will eventually concede that walking a 12-minute mile burns more calories than walking slower, but you can be sure that some will argue that most people can't and won't walk that fast. If the reputable sources of exercise information keep repeating that walking isn't intense and that walking faster isn't important, why will people ever try? The caloric-expenditure benefit of increased walking intensity is one of the best-kept secrets in the exercise field.

If the exercising public ever finds out about walking's intensity benefits for aerobic fitness and caloric expenditure, everyone, including the experts, will be amazed at how many people can walk faster than they thought possible. I am a living example of that. I am writing this section on March 4, 1991. It is an unusually warm, sunny day, and I have just returned from my 5-mile walk over country roads, of which 4 miles are rolling hills. At 63 years of age, I walked it in 55 minutes and 37 seconds, with plenty of speed to spare.

Do I walk this fast every day? Of course not. Tomorrow it might take me an hour to walk the same course. I walk at the speed I feel like each day. Even so, I usually do it at a pace of 12-minute miles or less. I am not a race walker; I walk only for weight control and cardiovascular fitness. But because I know I can burn more calories in less time by walking fast, I do it and enjoy it. Now that you know that speed really pays off by burning extra calories and reducing exercise time, maybe you will want to walk faster also. Physical exercise is exactly like mental exercise: you get out of it what you put into it.

When you are thinking about walking intensity in relation to energy expenditure, remember that any other exercise that supposedly will burn more calories in less time must be done at a very vigorous rate far more challenging than walking at a 12-minute-mile pace. What exercise can you expect to do vigorously four to seven days a week for a lifetime *except* walking? Review the seven exercise criteria in Chapter 7, and you will wonder how any other exercise for weight loss could be recommended over walking.

THE WEIGHT-LOSS PLATEAU

You are walking six days a week and eating a low-fat diet. The weight is coming off slowly but surely and you are pleased with your program. After, say, 20 pounds, the weight loss abruptly stops, even though you continue to do all the right things. This is the moment of truth called the weight-loss plateau. It reminds me of the "stitch in the side" phenomenon, because it doesn't happen to everybody, and why it happens is not easily explained.

Unfortunately, a weight-loss plateau causes a great number of people to throw in the towel if it lasts very long. Usually they end up saying, "Exercise doesn't work." (For some reason exercise seems to get blamed more than diet.) The September 1990 issue of

Weight Watchers' *Women's Health and Fitness News* discussed this troublesome aspect of weight loss and made the point that these plateaus can last "weeks, months, even up to a year."

Dr. Reva Frankle wrote: "Although the physiological causes of plateaus have not been fully studied the phenomena is a protective mechanism. . . . Faced with an ongoing caloric deficit that it interprets as starvation rather than safe dieting, the body puts on its brakes—and weight loss stops." For many this brings about a crisis of confidence and, all too often, a weakening of wills.

The story of Dianne Anderson, a young music teacher from Forest Park, Georgia, is the most extraordinary example of willpower on a weight-loss plateau that I have ever encountered. Dianne's story was told in the October 1990 issue of *Prevention*, a magazine that encourages exercise walking and conducts an annual national walkers' rally attended by thousands. More than any other, this fine magazine consistently promotes low-fat eating and exercise walking. Dianne's story will give you an idea of how long a plateau can last. More important, if you hit one, think of Dianne's will to win.

Dianne started at 321 pounds, with blood pressure that was out of sight. Over three and a half years she lost 184 pounds; her present weight is 137, and her blood pressure is now normal. She did it by a combination of exercise walking and a low-fat diet. After numerous failed attempts on her own, she and a friend started attending Weight Watchers. She received the counseling she needed for slow weight loss on a nutritional low-fat diet. The accountability of weighing in each week added to her commitment.

When she had lost 50 pounds by dieting alone, Dianne realized that she had so much more to lose that she would have to exercise, so she started exercise walking with the encouragement of her friend. (Unless you are extremely disciplined, exercise walking with a friend or a spouse is almost a prerequisite. Try to hook up with another overweight walker for peer support.)

In the first year, Dianne lost exactly 100 pounds, which brought her down to 221. Then came the dreaded weight-loss plateau, and in the next year she lost only 30 pounds. At one point she went four months without losing a pound. She plateaued at around 200 pounds, a weight that most women don't even reach. Dianne said, "I knew what I wanted to do, and that my body was having to make adjustments. I clung to the fact that I wasn't going to stop eating the healthy way I was eating whether I lost weight or not. I was committed to eating that way for the rest of my life."

Dianne's walking was critical in bringing her through this crisis. It had given her confidence in herself that she had not had before. When she started walking, she weighed 270 pounds and walked for an hour at a time at whatever pace she could manage. She generally was able to go about 3 miles. "But," she said, "gradually I started going faster, till I could get in 4 miles. Then I didn't worry about trying to walk any farther; I just started walking faster."

On June 26, 1991, I spoke with Dianne, who now lives in Tempe, Arizona. She said that she still walks 4 miles a day, five days a week, for weight maintenance. She usually covers the distance in about 48 minutes, an average pace of 12 minutes per mile. From a snail's-pace beginning she is now burning up the roads— and the calories. Her combination of desire and discipline to conquer that four-month weight-loss plateau is truly remarkable.

MAINTAINING WEIGHT LOSS: THE TOUGHEST CHALLENGE

For many, getting the weight off is less of a challenge than *keeping* it off. Oprah Winfrey found this out, to her bitter disappointment. She told *People* that losing her excess weight was "the single greatest accomplishment in my life." Sadly, Oprah psyched herself up to lose weight quickly without firmly committing to the rules of permanent weight loss. Even before the program was over, she dropped out of her group, abandoned the maintenance program, and quit exercising, according to *People*. Remember the old margarine commercial that said, "You can't fool Mother Nature"? This saying was never more true than when applied to losing weight and keeping it off. The rules for success are clear, and there are no shortcuts.

Dianne Anderson took three and a half years to lose 184 pounds, with one whole year a heartbreaker. This may have been the test of fire that prepared her mentally and physically to control her weight for the rest of her life. The ability to ride out delays and setbacks in a weight-loss program galvanizes individual resolve.

In the final analysis, weight maintenance is a mind-set that must take over after the biological battle to lose the weight has been won. In the October 1990 issue of *Women's Health and Fitness News*, Carol Morton, senior program developer at Weight Watchers, said: "Weight maintenance is a decision that has to be made early in a weight-control program—consciously and with commitment. . . . It goes beyond the dieting mentality, where the focus is on losing. In fact, reaching one's goal weight is really the beginning, not the end." That is probably the difference between Oprah and Dianne. Oprah thought she was "cured," but Dianne knew better. The surest way to guaranteed weight maintenance is a strong, consistent exercise-walking program. Long-term exercisers are long-term weight controllers.

As pointed out earlier, exercise of any kind requires a time commitment and physical effort, whereas dieting does not. For those who don't have a full grasp of the importance of exercise, there is a tendency to shorten it with the mental note to make up the caloric difference by dieting a little harder that day. Unfortunately, these kinds of lapses never work out.

Weight maintenance is most difficult for career women who are also raising families. I visit with them in my walking clinics, and the demands of meals, laundry, dishes, cleaning, kids, and husbands (who they tell me are often more trouble than the kids), coupled with a full-time job, make finding time for exercise nearly impossible. Yet where there's a will there's a way. At an evening clinic I held in Houston a few years ago, I met Terri, a 33-year-old mother of two who works full-time as a paralegal. She told me that without her walking program she is convinced that she would gain back the 28 pounds she worked so hard to lose after the birth of her second baby. This was exactly what happened to her after the birth of her first child, when she tried to keep her weight off with diet alone.

Terri is organized and committed, and she makes sure that she gets in 2 hours of walking every Saturday and Sunday. Three days a week she is at the nearby shopping mall when the doors open at 6:00 A.M. She walks 45 minutes at a fast pace, then returns home before 7:00 to get herself and her family off for the day.

Although Terri's schedule may seem exhausting, she said the walking actually elevates her energy level. After her first baby was born, when she didn't exercise, she was always logy and tired. Elevated energy level is common to all exercise walkers, and it becomes an important contribution to weight maintenance. You do not see many highly active, energetic people who are fat. With a mind-set and a game plan, Terri is now in control of her weight. As I bade her good-bye at the end of my clinic, she said, "I have to confess that some days it isn't easy." Then she smiled and added, "But anything really worthwhile rarely is."

TO WEIGH OR NOT TO WEIGH

A number of experts in the weight loss field recommend that you weigh yourself only once a week. This is a judgment call based mostly on the fact that your weight doesn't actually change much on a daily basis but that your water weight may. If you happen to eat some highly salted food, for instance, you may show a gain of a pound or two overnight. The reasoning for weighing yourself once a week is that a sudden jump may cause you to get unwarrantedly discouraged.

I will give you the rationale why Carol and I weigh ourselves every day, and why we write our weights down. First, however, it is important to have good scales. For a few dollars more than the little digital scales, which aren't very accurate, you can buy a doctor's type scale with weights that slide back and forth on a bar. But whether digital or doctor's type, the scale should always be on a level, hard surface. Carpeting can cause you to get an erroneous reading.

When weighing every day, it is important to weigh at exactly the same time, because your weight will fluctuate, depending on food and liquid intake. Carol and I weigh ourselves when we get up every morning, immediately after our toilet duties and before any intake of food or water. Our scale and clipboard with pencil are nearby. In the buff, we weigh ourselves and write our weights down next to the day's date. I never weigh at any other time of the day, and on those rare occasions when I am in a hurry and forget to do so in the morning, I don't bother until the next morning.

Weighing first thing in the morning and writing your weight down is helpful for two reasons. First, you get a consistent tracking of what your weight *really* is. Secondly, the fact that you know what it is each day means you have made a mental note of it before any of the day's distractions. I promise you that your weight will keep coming back to haunt you like a bad check at every temptation to stray from your calorie counting or exercise plan.

Since my weight hasn't fluctuated 2 pounds in eight years, why do I weigh myself every day? Well, perhaps that's why it hasn't fluctuated. Because I am always aware of my weight, I am also always aware of what my options are. Sometimes they let me eat something that I might not otherwise indulge in, like a couple of bites of a tempting dessert.

Another benefit of daily weighing is to familiarize yourself with your weight fluctuations. If you know why they occur, you won't push the panic button every time your weight jumps a pound or two. During the writing of this chapter, Carol and I went to dinner at our favorite Chinese restaurant with some friends. The next morning my weight was up 1¼ pounds. I shrugged it off because it always jumps like that when I eat at a Chinese restaurant. It is all water retention from salt, not fat, and in a day or two I am back to my regular weight.

Knowing more about your weight fluctuations seems to me to be a much better way to control your weight after you have reached your goal. You will soon know whether the scale is weighing water or new fat. For instance, if your weight jumps a pound overnight, think back on what you ate and drank in the preceding 24 hours. Do a mental calculation to see if you actually consumed 3,500 more calories than you normally do. Unless you were involved in an unusual pig out, which you would certainly remember, that extra pound is probably mostly water. The more you know about your body and how it functions, the better armed you are to make the right decisions about diet and exercise.

DON'T SMORGASBORD YOUR EXERCISE DURING WEIGHT LOSS

In my walking clinics with people trying to lose weight I ask, "How many here would like to lose your excess weight as quickly as possible?" Without exception, every hand goes up. I have two reasons for asking the question: (1) to remind everyone that "as quickly as possible" actually means losing only about a pound or less per week if you are going to do it the healthy, sustainable way; (2) to tell them why exercise walking should be their *only* exercise during their weight-loss period.

As I write this, I can already feel the vibrations from exercise physiologists. What about running, cycling, swimming, rowing machines, aerobics classes, and what about muscle toning? My answer is, What about them? In the first place, if people don't lose their weight, they won't stay with any of those exercises; in the second place, some of those exercises don't contribute anything to accelerating weight loss, and some may even delay it. Few people know that *not all exercises contribute to weight loss*. Starting with the premise that you also want to lose weight as quickly as possible, or have already lost weight and want to keep it off, I'll show you why walking is the only exercise you really need.

Swimming has often been mentioned as an aerobic exercise and as good for cardiovascular fitness. Certainly for arthritics who may suffer pain working against gravity, it may be the only option. If you can walk, however, swimming should not be your exercise for weight loss. A study published in the *Tufts University Diet and Nutrition Letter* was conducted at the University of California, Irvine, Medical Center in which three groups of overweight women exercised daily for six months by walking, cycling, or swimming. The swimmers actually gained an average of 5 pounds, while the walkers lost an average of 17 pounds and the cyclists a similar amount. Just as important, the body fat on the swimmers, measured by skin-fold thickness, did not change, whereas the body fat on the walkers and cyclists dropped considerably.

The comparison of other exercises and walking in Chapter 7 cited a study indicating that swimming increases the appetite. If you are on a weight-loss program, this is like throwing an anchor to a drowning man. In the Tufts report, Dr. Grant Gwinup, who monitored the study, speculated that swimmers eat more to compensate for the calories they burn because water draws more heat away from the body than air. Swimmers' bodies sense this extra heat loss, which stimulates their appetites so that they can hold on to the layers of fat that serve as heat-preserving "insulation."

The Tufts letter reported that Dr. Gwinup's theory is strengthened by the fact that people who spend a lot of time in the water maintain body fat particularly well. Polynesians, for instance, who are in the water comparatively often, and Japanese women pearl divers have high body-fat ratios. Ultradistance swimmers, like those who swim the English Channel, also carry a considerable amount of body fat. Swimming versus walking for weight loss doesn't look like a good choice.

Cycling may be okay as a way to burn calories, but when I look at some of the people in my classes at the Cooper Wellness Program who are in their 40s, 50s, and 60s and who are 30 to 60 pounds overweight, I wonder, on a risk-reward basis, whether cycling should ever be recommended over walking. To burn many calories, a cyclist has to get up a pretty good head of steam—about 15 miles per hour. A 50-year-old cyclist who is 40 pounds overweight—and there are a lot of them—would make quite a splash if he or she fell at that speed. Stacked up against the seven criteria for the perfect exercise, cycling can't compare with walking for weight loss.

Chapter 7 registered my disdain for the overadvertised, over-promoted exercise equipment, such as exercise cycles, rowing machines, stair climbers, and others. For any of this equipment to have much effect on weight loss, the exerciser has to use it with considerable intensity over an extended period. The cumulative, boring effect of this unnatural activity soon leads to exercise burnout.

Many exercise experts advise muscle toning during the weight-loss period. Ostensibly this is to strengthen and tighten your muscles while you are losing your flab. In theory it makes sense, but in practicality it may be a waste of time and actually delay weight loss. Muscle toning may not even be necessary if you lose your weight by walking intensively.

I find many people don't know that lifting weights or working out on weight-resistance equipment like Nautilus does not burn calories aerobically. Consequently people trying to peel off excess pounds are actually *delaying* their weight loss by spending their exercise time on muscle-building equipment.

Here is my personal recommendation and experience with muscle toning. During the weight-loss period, spend every minute of your time doing an aerobic exercise that uses the most major muscle groups and burns the most calories per minute. Obviously I am talking about walking. Start at a stroll, and simply keep increasing the frequency, duration, and intensity. Once you reach the weight you want to be, *then* take a good look at yourself. Where exactly are you flabby? How much muscle toning do you truly need?

If you lost your weight by walking, and especially if you worked up to the aerobic 12-minute-mile pace, I guarantee that from the waist down you will be firm. If you are an aerobic walker, your chest, shoulders, and back muscles will also have good muscle tone. The only thing a walker doesn't develop are big biceps. Decide if you really want them after you have reached your weight goal.

Except for doing 14 push-ups three or four days a week, the

only exercise I do is walk, but, as you know by now, I walk at a pretty good clip. My legs are hard as rocks, and my upper body is shaped like a swimmer's from all my vigorous arm swinging. At my last physical at the Cooper Clinic, on November 1, 1990, my body fat was only 16 percent. I do no muscle toning, because pumping iron or its equivalent doesn't appeal to me.

Much of the misconception about how you can flatten your stomach comes from highly promoted contraptions promising to help you get rid of your flab. They range from springs that you hook over your feet and pull on to big, thick rubber bands to pull on. The unsuspecting public assumes that "flab" means fat, not flabby muscles. Spot reducing is a dead issue; don't waste your time trying it, and don't waste your money on some springs or rubber bands in the hope that they will make your stomach look like the one in the ad. If you are carrying a spare tire, your only option is to go to work and use up the excess fat that you have stored around your waist. This calls for walking, and lots of it.

The July 25, 1988, issue of *USA Today* had a cover story about a 10-year-old girl trying to lose 52 pounds. It described in glowing terms how a fitness center for kids in Virginia had structured a weight-loss exercise program for this youngster. It was the worst case of exercise smorgasbording that I have ever encountered. The poor child, who had a serious weight problem, was pictured working out on a weight-lifting machine! She had lost 12 pounds, according to the article, but still had 40 more to lose. "So the bright 10 year old, a veteran of many failed diets, signed up for a special fitness program two months ago," the writer gushed. A "veteran of many failed diets" at only 10 years of age! Sadly, she was about to become a failed exercise veteran as well, which at her tender age will undoubtedly turn her against exercise for many years, if not for life.

According to the article, the girl's exercise program to lose weight included "riding a stationary bike, weight training, using a rowing machine, jogging and playing games." By my count only one out of those five has any long-term merit as exercise for a 10-year-old girl. Games are fun at 10 years of age, and, while they may not be aerobic, they will at least keep this girl active and interested. Exercise equipment is a quick burnout for adults and has no chance at all with kids. According to *USA Today*, the child said, "I don't like running, but I have to do it for my program so I am starting to like it more." When a 10-year-old says, "I have to do it," she is simply saying that some adult has told her this is her medicine and she has to take it. When it comes to exercise, whether they are 10 or 60 years old, people will not do something they don't like for long.

The heading of the story's continuation read "Make Sure It's Fun." Does anyone reading this story think that what I have just told you would be fun if *you* were an overweight 10-year-old? Would it even be fun at the age you are now? How in the world could an exercise cycle, rowing machine, weight machine, and jogging be fun for a 10-year-old?

The most obvious flaw in this weight-loss program was the total absence of walking. Those young legs and young lungs are ideally suited for bent-arm-swing aerobic walking. Hook a Walkman onto her with some of her favorite rock music, and this young girl could burn a lot of calories every day while truly having fun. More important, when she is 40 she will still be walking. There is no chance at all that she'll be jogging or using an exercise cycle or rowing machine.

For a struggling 10-year-old or a famous celebrity like Oprah Winfrey, the solution to weight loss and weight maintenance is the same. The importance of exercise is undeniable, and the importance of walking as the most effective, sustainable exercise of all is equally undeniable. I have been accused of being overzealous about exercise walking. Maybe I am, but what a wonderful thing to be overzealous about. When you measure it against all the other recommended exercises, it is in a class by itself.

Whether you are about to embark on a weight-loss program or are struggling to maintain the weight you now have, exercise walking at an intensity level that you can attain consistently should become as important to you as bathing or brushing your teeth. Embrace it as part of your daily life-style, not as a dreaded dose of exercise medicine. You will enjoy walking, and you will enjoy even more the confidence of knowing that you have your weight problem under control permanently.

It doesn't matter if you are as obese as Dianne Anderson was. Start walking as she did, slowly but consistently. Remember that walking is not a bridge to a more vigorous exercise, walking is a bridge to a happier, healthier life. If you want a more vigorous exercise, all you have to do is walk faster. Walking is the complete exercise.

But as convinced and as enthused as I am about walking as the exercise solution to everyone's weight problem, it is still only half of the equation. Walking will provide the energy expenditure part of the weight equation. The energy intake part must come not from diet (as in denial), but from what I call eating smart.

13

EATING SMART, LIVING LEAN, AND LIVING LONGER

There's an old saying that "man is the only animal who eats when he is not hungry, drinks when he is not thirsty, and has sex in all seasons." Only one of these three isn't fattening. I have covered exercise and its importance in previous chapters but, as I pointed out in the last one, it is only half of the weight-control equation. The equally important half is diet—not diet as *denial* but diet as in the composition of daily food intake. It was the combination of exercise and a low-fat, high-complex-carbohydrate diet that enabled me to stabilize my weight exactly where I wanted it after years of losing and gaining, losing and gaining.

The purpose of this chapter is to alert you to the dietary pitfalls facing every unknowing, unsuspecting weight-conscious person, and to show you how easy it is to eat smart. Learning a few things, such as how many calories are in a gram of fat and how to read a food label, will help you immensely to control your weight. Once you learn to figure the amount of fat in food as a percent of its total calories, you will have the information you need to control your daily fat intake. Notice that I said *fat* intake, not calorie intake. If you control your fat calories, your total calorie intake will start to level off and should not be a major problem as long as you exercise.

FINDING OUT ABOUT FAT

At the start of my walking clinics, I always ask how many people are on a diet to lose weight or are carefully watching what they eat so that they won't gain weight. The show of hands is usually 50 percent or more. I immediately emphasize that they can't walk enough miles to control their weight unless they are eating smart, and then I ask, How many calories are in a gram of fat? Generally less than 25 percent of the women know and *none* of the men unless they happen to be in the food industry or a related business.

I don't believe anybody who has a weight problem can control his weight over the long term if he does not know how many fat calories he consumes each day. All exercises are not equal for weight control, and all calories are not either. Your body will not handle 100 calories of fat in the same way it will handle 100 calories of complex carbohydrates. Consequently, cutting fat calories becomes your number one dietary priority for long-term weight control and a healthier heart.

The body processes fat calories and carbohydrate calories differently, and, according to Dr. Bryant M. Stamford, in a May 1990 article in *The Physician and Sportsmedicine*, the body easily converts dietary fat to body fat. This conversion process uses only 3 calories per 100 calories of fat consumed, meaning that 97 fat calories out of 100 can be stored as body fat. And there's a wrinkle you may not be aware of. According to Dr. Stamford, "Fat storage is accelerated when you consume fat and simple sugar at the same meal—combining a sugared cola and french fries, for example. . . . Sugar triggers the release of insulin and insulin activates fat-cell enzymes which promote the passage of fat from the bloodstream into fat cells."

A shift to more intake of complex carbohydrates (vegetables, fruits, legumes, and grains) can reduce fat storage even when you don't reduce your calorie intake. According to Dr. Stamford, this is true for three reasons. The first is that carbohydrates can be stored as glycogen, which prevents their conversion to fat. Even though glycogen storage is limited, Dr. Stamford said, "The body can expand storage capacity in those who regularly consume large amounts of carbohydrates and in those who exercise regularly."

The second reason is that, when maximum storage capacity is reached, the body increases its metabolic rate to burn off excess carbohydrates. Third, there's a bit of a safety valve when storage and increased metabolism are inadequate to handle the carbohydrate load and the body has to convert the excess to fat. Dr. Stamford pointed out that this conversion process is calorically costly; it requires 23 calories of every 100 calories of carbohydrates consumed. This means that only 77 out of 100 would be stored as fat.

These three factors ensure that "less body fat results from carbohydrate calories than from an equal number of fat calories," Dr. Stamford wrote. "The bottom line: if optimal health and slender physique are your goals, a low-fat, high-carbohydrate diet coupled with mild, comfortable exercise will accomplish much more than vigorous exercise coupled with a high-fat diet." It will help you to live lean.

Living leaner is relative, however, and will not be the same for everyone. Genes play a big part in how lean you can expect to be. If you were lucky enough to have tall, slender parents, you will have a tendency to be like them, and fat may not be a problem no matter what you eat. If you have stocky parents or grandparents who tended to be fat, then you must wrestle with genes that will probably make weight control an unending problem. It need not be an unmanageable one, however. By reducing fat intake and by walking every day, a person who has such a genetic tendency can maintain his or her weight within a healthy range.

The magic number to remember is 9. There are 9 calories in 1 gram of fat, and all food labels list fat in grams. There are only 4 calories in a gram of carbohydrates, so ounce for ounce or gram for gram you get less than half the calories per serving of equal weight.

Before we go any further, let's establish the relationship of ounces and pounds to grams. Here is an easy guide to help you read nutrition labels:

1 pound (lb) = 454 grams (g)
1 ounce (oz) = 28 grams (g)
1 gram (g) = 1,000 milligrams (mg)
1 milligram (mg) = 1,000 micrograms (mcg)

On food labels, the key equivalence to remember is that 1 ounce = 28 grams. To get a perspective on relative weight, 1 gram is about what a paper clip weighs.

You've probably heard the old trick question What weighs more, a pound of lead or a pound of feathers? Although they weigh the same, it is not a trick question when I ask, Which one takes up the most room? Obviously, the weight density of lead makes it smaller. Using a similar comparison question, Which takes up the most room, 500 calories of fat or 500 calories of complex carbohydrates? The 9-to-4 ratio makes fat much denser. A small portion of food high in fat can pack a lot of calories per ounce, which makes it easier to eat more of it than you should. Portion control is vital for fat control.

Kathy Duran is the registered dietitian who teaches Cooper Wellness Program participants everything they need to know about low-fat eating, low-fat cooking, how to shop for low-fat foods, and how to stock a low-fat kitchen. I have eaten many of her delicious lunches and dinners that have less than 20 percent fat in them. She's a whiz as a teacher and a cook and is the source for much of the information in this chapter.

If you are going to regulate your fat intake, it's important to know that there are three kinds of fat: saturated, monounsaturated (*mono* meaning "one"), and polyunsaturated (*poly* meaning "many"). From a cholesterol standpoint, saturated fat is the one that the American Heart Association recommends you limit to 10 percent *or less* of your calories. It is found primarily in red meat, but poultry and fish also have some. Palm oil, palm kernel oil, and coconut oil are heavy with it. Avoid them. It is important to remember, however, that, while the other two fats are not harmful from a cholesterol standpoint, all three fats have the same number of calories: 9 per gram. All three are equally fattening.

The typical American diet averages between 40 and 50 percent fat calories, but the American Heart Association recommends that you reduce your fat-calorie intake to 30 percent *or less* of your total calories. There is some growing speculation that even 30 percent fat may be too much for the long term. Certainly reducing your fat intake to 20 percent or less will help you reach your weight goal more quickly and more safely.

If you want to go on a 1,500-calorie diet and want to know what 30 percent fat calories amounts to, here is a simple example:

$$1,500 \text{ calories} \times 0.30 = 450 \text{ calories from fat}$$
$$450 \text{ calories} \div 9 = 50 \text{ grams of fat}$$

Reducing the diet to 20 percent fat calories would go like this:

$$1,500 \text{ calories} \times 0.20 = 300 \text{ calories from fat}$$
$$300 \text{ calories} \div 9 = 33.3 \text{ grams of fat}$$

Fat grams for other amounts of total caloric intake can be figured using the same formula.

Since we are not accustomed to thinking in terms of grams, it is difficult to visualize what 50.0 or 33.3 grams of fat amounts to in our daily food intake. The March 1991 issue of the *University of California at Berkeley Wellness Letter* listed some commonly eaten foods that would overshoot 50.0 fat grams a day and double 33.3. Some portions are fairly large, but most are not. For example:

Double-stuffed sandwich cookies (10) and
  1 cup whole milk—42 grams
Salad dressing, commercial (6 tablespoons)—54 grams
Cheese (5 ounces) and high-fat crackers (10)—55 grams
Fried chicken, fast-food, 1 breast, 1 drumstick
  and 1 wing—55 grams
Cheesecake (2 average 4-ounce slices)—56 grams
Cheese enchiladas (2) and refried beans—60 grams
Porterhouse steak, untrimmed (10 ounces, cooked)—63 grams
Large fast-food hamburger, large fries, shake—64 grams
Pork sausage (three 2.5-ounce links)—65 grams
Peanuts, oil-roasted (1 cup)—71 grams
Potato chips (8-ounce bag)—80 grams
Superpremium ice cream, butter pecan (1 pint)—96 grams

I look at that list and think back over how many times I have eaten a 16- or 20-ounce porterhouse steak. In the old days, 10 ounces was the "ladies' portion." I can inhale a cup of warm, salted cashew nuts in about 8 minutes, and a pint of butter pecan ice cream was just a normal portion. Is it any wonder I ballooned 52 pounds and four suit sizes? Those days are gone forever, and I don't miss them at all.

Now, eating small portions of fat foods and large portions of complex carbohydrates, which digest quickly, I have a high energy level, no weight problem, and feel brand-new at the age of 64. So will you if you kick the fat habit and convert at least 60 percent of your caloric intake to complex carbohydrates, 15 percent to protein, and only 25 percent or less to fat.

Throughout this book I have said that one can't generalize about the human animal. However, I have not found anyone who doesn't feel that quality of life, state of health, and general well-being wasn't better once he or she got off heavy fat foods and started exercising. Once you turn the corner and quit letting sweet, fat food dominate your life, you will wonder why you didn't do it sooner.

THE TRICKY FOOD LABELS

If you really want to reduce your fat intake, perhaps the biggest unexpected obstacle you will face will be some of the major food companies in the United States. They have found that rich, sweet, fat, oversalted food appeals to more taste buds than more healthful, less sweetened, low-fat, lower-sodium food. Obviously they are going to put on the grocery shelves what sells the best. You have to be able to sort out the junk foods from the nutritious, wholesome, healthful foods. You must learn how to read food labels.

Kathy Duran says surveys reveal that Americans will spend up to 33 percent more for a product with the word *natural* on the label. Are you aware of the many other nutritional buzzwords that food processors print prominently on their brightly colored packages? For instance, suppose you saw an attractively colored box on the grocery store shelf with the following in big letters: "Low-calorie, low-fat, low-sodium, no cholesterol, no sugar added, no preservatives, no additives, no artificial coloring, high fiber, and 100% natural." Sounds like the perfect health food, doesn't it? Be careful, though; it could also be a box of horse manure. Don't get taken in by the nutritional buzzwords.

The information you really need will probably be in the small print near the bottom on the side or back of the package. This is usually where you find the nutrition label, which contains information required by the Food and Drug Administration (FDA) and the U.S. Department of Agriculture (USDA), plus information supplied at the option of the food processor. This is where you find out how much fat is really in the product.

FIGURE 13.1
Breakdown of a food label for yogurt raisins

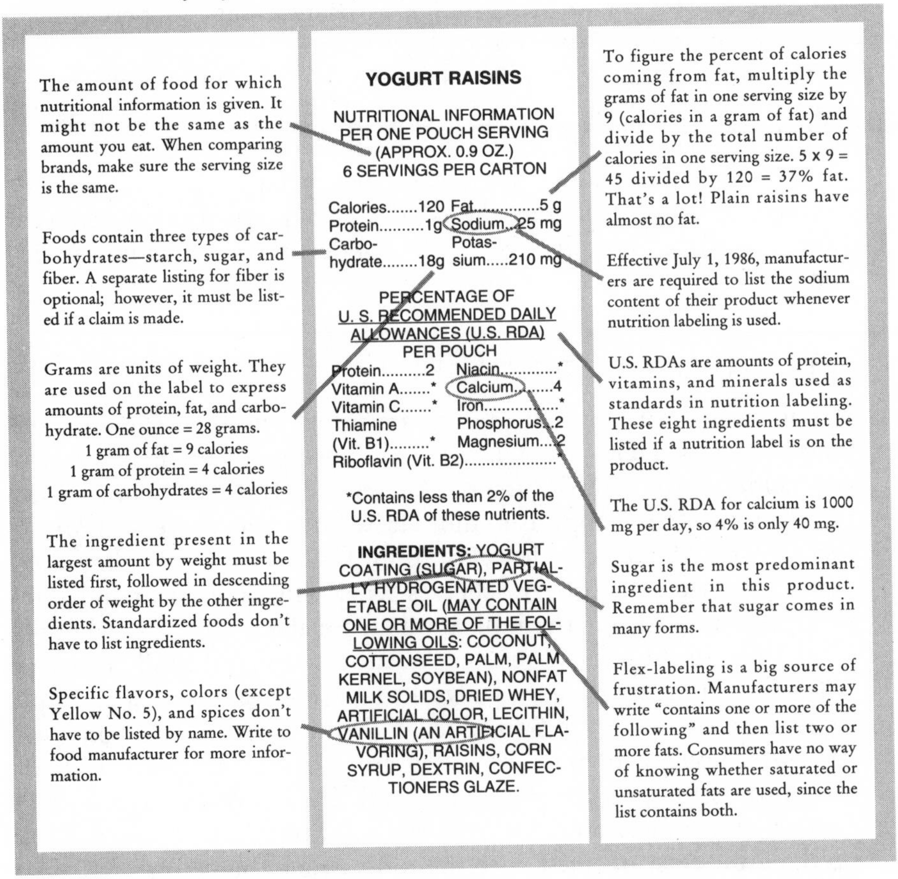

The amount of food for which nutritional information is given. It might not be the same as the amount you eat. When comparing brands, make sure the serving size is the same.

Foods contain three types of carbohydrates—starch, sugar, and fiber. A separate listing for fiber is optional; however, it must be listed if a claim is made.

Grams are units of weight. They are used on the label to express amounts of protein, fat, and carbohydrate. One ounce = 28 grams.
1 gram of fat = 9 calories
1 gram of protein = 4 calories
1 gram of carbohydrates = 4 calories

The ingredient present in the largest amount by weight must be listed first, followed in descending order of weight by the other ingredients. Standardized foods don't have to list ingredients.

Specific flavors, colors (except Yellow No. 5), and spices don't have to be listed by name. Write to food manufacturer for more information.

YOGURT RAISINS

NUTRITIONAL INFORMATION
PER ONE POUCH SERVING
(APPROX. 0.9 OZ.)
6 SERVINGS PER CARTON

Calories......120 Fat............5 g
Protein..........1g Sodium...25 mg
Carbo-   Potas-
hydrate........18g sium.....210 mg

PERCENTAGE OF
U. S. RECOMMENDED DAILY
ALLOWANCES (U.S. RDA)
PER POUCH
Protein..........2 Niacin............*
Vitamin A.......* Calcium.....4
Vitamin C.......* Iron............*
Thiamine   Phosphorus..2
(Vit. B1).........* Magnesium...2
Riboflavin (Vit. B2)....................

*Contains less than 2% of the
U.S. RDA of these nutrients.

INGREDIENTS: YOGURT
COATING (SUGAR), PARTIAL-
LY HYDROGENATED VEG-
ETABLE OIL (MAY CONTAIN
ONE OR MORE OF THE FOL-
LOWING OILS: COCONUT,
COTTONSEED, PALM, PALM
KERNEL, SOYBEAN), NONFAT
MILK SOLIDS, DRIED WHEY,
ARTIFICIAL COLOR, LECITHIN,
VANILLIN (AN ARTIFICIAL FLA-
VORING), RAISINS, CORN
SYRUP, DEXTRIN, CONFEC-
TIONERS GLAZE.

To figure the percent of calories coming from fat, multiply the grams of fat in one serving size by 9 (calories in a gram of fat) and divide by the total number of calories in one serving size. 5 x 9 = 45 divided by 120 = 37% fat. That's a lot! Plain raisins have almost no fat.

Effective July 1, 1986, manufacturers are required to list the sodium content of their product whenever nutrition labeling is used.

U.S. RDAs are amounts of protein, vitamins, and minerals used as standards in nutrition labeling. These eight ingredients must be listed if a nutrition label is on the product.

The U.S. RDA for calcium is 1000 mg per day, so 4% is only 40 mg.

Sugar is the most predominant ingredient in this product. Remember that sugar comes in many forms.

Flex-labeling is a big source of frustration. Manufacturers may write "contains one or more of the following" and then list two or more fats. Consumers have no way of knowing whether saturated or unsaturated fats are used, since the list contains both.

Under current FDA regulations, any food to which a nutrient has been added, or any food for which a nutrition claim is made, must have its nutritional content listed on the label. Nutrition labels tell you how many calories and how many grams of protein, carbohydrates, and fat are in a serving of the product. The labels also list the percentages of the U.S. recommended daily allowances (U.S. RDAs) of protein and 7 important vitamins and minerals in each serving. Finally, the labels tell you the size of a serving (for example, 1 cup, 2 ounces, 1 tablespoon), and how many servings there are in the container. The listing of 12 other vitamins and minerals and of cholesterol, fatty acid, and sodium content is optional.

Figure 13.1 is an easily understood breakdown of a food label for Yogurt Raisins that Kathy Duran uses in her classes. Note that the ingredient in the largest amount by weight must be listed first, followed in descending order by weight of the other ingredients.

The box in the lower-right-hand corner addresses flex labeling. This means the company can give you a list of ingredients that may or may not be in the product. The example here of the vegetable oils—coconut, cottonseed, palm, palm kernel, and soybean—is the flex label to be most cautious about. All these oils have 100 percent fat calories, but the tropical oils—coconut, palm, and palm kernel—are extremely high in saturated fat, which may adversely affect your cholesterol level.

Never buy a product that flex-labels the tropical oils if you must control your cholesterol level. If the company expects you to guess which oils it is using, always assume it is using the wrong ones. You can certainly bet it is using the lowest-priced oil. As this chapter was being written, I checked *The Wall Street Journal*'s list of the cash price of commodities. It showed soybean oil (a good vegetable oil) at 22 cents a pound, palm oil at 19 cents a pound, and coconut oil at 16 cents a pound. Guess which oil is in a flex-labeled product that lists those three.

Grocery store aisles are filled with caloric land mines. Tiptoeing through them to buy the right kinds of healthful foods is a nutritional game of wits. You must take the position that many food companies are more interested in your wallet than in your waistline. If it's in a box, bottle, jar, or package and doesn't have a complete nutritional food label on it telling me how many fat grams are in it, I don't buy it—and neither should you. If a flex label lists any ingredient you shouldn't be eating, don't buy the product. Always look for a product that is fully labeled so you can make a buying decision based on proper nutritional information. However, this may be easier said than done.

The Fat Sandwich

The October 1987 issue of the *Tufts University Diet and Nutrition Letter* waded through some of the labeling double-talk that food processors use. In particular, it examined the luncheon meats, deli meats, and cold cuts in those little see-through packages that you find on the pegboards above supermarket meat counters.

The convenience of sliced, packaged lunch meats comes at a very high fat-caloric price per serving, but the companies selling you this stuff do all kinds of mathematical gyrations to make you believe otherwise. They start with the portion size. It is usually a 1-ounce slice. When was the last time you made a cold-cut sandwich and used only one slice? By breaking the calories down into small increments, the meat processors focus your mind on a small number while you are piling on four or five slices to make a tasty sandwich.

The article pointed out that a ¾-ounce slice of Oscar Mayer's "95 percent fat free smoked, cooked ham with natural juices" contains 8 calories of fat out of a total of 23 calories. Logically you would expect it to have only 5 percent fat calories if something is "95 percent fat free." Don't believe it, because it isn't so. In the fat-calorie shell game, the phrase "95 percent fat free" means that the remaining 5 percent is fat by weight, not by calories. Therefore the 8 fat calories in this tiny portion actually represent 35 percent fat. Thirty-five percent fat is pretty low for lunch meat, but by the time you get four or five of those slices on a sandwich, with maybe a slice of cheese and some mayonnaise (all of which contain large amounts of fat), the sandwich isn't as fat free as you think.

In the past decade, the emphasis on meat has swung from beef and pork to poultry as a healthier choice from the standpoint of cholesterol and saturated fat. White meat without the skin from a turkey breast is considered the lowest in cholesterol and saturated fat. This part of the turkey has only about 18 percent fat calories. Louis Rich sells packaged turkey breasts that are cooked and ready to eat. Carol and I use them all the time, and they are delicious. But what do they do with the rest of the turkey? They make turkey bologna, turkey salami, and turkey pastrami out of it. Judging from the fat numbers on those products, they must throw in everything, including the gobble.

Don't get caught up in the fat numbers game with processed turkey, because you can end up with just as much fat as is in a piece of regular bologna or salami. The Tufts article letter revealed that a Louis Rich 1-ounce "82 percent fat free" slice of turkey bologna has *73 percent fat calories*. By comparison, Oscar Mayer's beef bologna (without a "fat-free" pitch) has 84 percent fat calories. Once you get up into those high-fat numbers, the 11 percent difference between the two doesn't mean much—you've already blown it.

With meat processors, if it isn't the numbers game with fat, then it's the word game. The March 1991 issue of the *University of California at Berkeley Wellness Letter* warns that meat labels deceptively use the words *lean*, *lite*, and *light* to imply that a brand is considerably lower in fat than the regular product. A few examples cited: Eckrich smoked or Polish sausage (regular), 1 ounce—85 percent calories by fat. Eckrich "lite" Polish sausage —77 percent fat calories. When you already have more than double the amount of fat you should be eating, what is 8 percent? *Sizzlean* has a nice ring to it, but a serving has 80 percent fat calories. Hillshire Farms' sausage (regular) is 81 percent fat calories, and the "lite" version is 76 percent. Big deal!

As you begin to alter the composition of your daily diet to get its fat content down below 30 percent, you might as well forget sausage and processed lunch meats. Almost all of this kind of meat has more than double the percentage of fat you should be eating, which means you would have to cut back severely on all your other fat intake.

I focus on meat because we are a nation of meat eaters—as compared with Asiatic countries, for instance, where rice is the main food. There small portions of meat, almost like a condiment, are added from time to time to rice dishes. In this country, however, the main course is usually a meat dish. If you can regulate your meat intake, you will be well on your way to mastering your fat-calorie intake.

In my view, the portion sizes used to calculate calories, cholesterol, and saturated fat content for *unprocessed* meat are also totally unrealistic. Those portions are *3 ounces*. Where can you order a 3-ounce steak? The petite filet mignon, the smallest, is 6 ounces in every restaurant I have patronized. Where in the supermarket are steaks cut and packaged in 4-ounce sizes (generally 4 ounces raw = 3 ounces cooked)?

According to a study, the average portion of meat eaten per meal is about 5.4 ounces. Consequently, when you see some celebrity in a TV commercial for the beef industry touting only 150 calories per 3-ounce serving, you may as well double that number for the real world. The same goes for poultry and pork. All of the numbers quoted are about half of what the average person eats at an average meal. It is this kind of impractical information that causes people to eat more fat than they realize—and more than they should.

Table 13.1 lists the calories, fat, saturated fat, and cholesterol in various cuts of beef, pork, and poultry. In this chart, too, the numbers given are for the unrealistic 3-ounce servings.

People are now eating more poultry to reduce cholesterol and saturated-fat intake. You may be kidding yourself, however, about fat intake if you don't eat the right piece and *skin it*. Look at the bottom number in the fat column: 9.47 grams of fat for 3 ounces of chicken drumstick meat with the skin. Now look at the other numbers in that column; your piece of chicken had *more* fat grams than any of the lean beef or pork. Notice also that a chicken breast with skin has more than double the fat grams of one without skin.

Choosing the right meat and watching the portion sizes are a good start. Kathy Duran advises avoiding "prime"-grade meats, heavily marbled or fatty cuts—for example, corned beef, bacon, pastrami, spareribs, short ribs, rib eye roast or steak, most ground meats, frankfurters, sausages, most lunch meats, goose, domestic duck, and organ meats, such as liver and sweetbreads. Organ meats are also the highest in cholesterol.

Kathy says that the best choices to reduce fat as a percentage of total calories and cholesterol are fish and shellfish (but that you should limit shrimp because of its high cholesterol content to no more than a couple of servings per week), along with chicken and turkey (particularly the white meat with all skin removed), lean beef, veal, pork, and lamb, trimmed of all visible fat. Limit red meat to a maximum of two or three servings per week, and have no more than 6 ounces of meat a day. Like me, you may struggle with this for a while. If you can turn the corner on meat consumption, you are on your way to a lifetime of weight control. If you doubt me, how many fat vegetarians do you know?

Kathy emphasizes that the leanest cut of meat can become a fat dish if it is cooked by the wrong method. Meat should never be fried. Baking, broiling, grilling, microwaving, and stir-frying in a wok with very small amounts of cooking oil are the most healthful, lowest-fat ways to prepare meat, so retire the frying pan.

Instant Math

Figuring fat as a percentage of total calories is fairly simple, yet I sometimes find myself in the grocery store trying to do instant math and becoming frustrated. The easiest way to compute it is shown in the top right-hand box in Figure 13.1. In addition, Kathy

TABLE 13.1.

Good choices for reducing fat and cholesterol

NAME OF CUT	CALORIES	FAT (grams)	SATURATED FAT (grams)	CHOLESTEROL (milligrams)
Beef (lean only, Choice grade)				
Top round steak, broiled	165	5.49	1.92	72
Eye of round, roasted	156	5.68	2.17	59
Tip round, roast	164	6.59	2.41	69
Sirloin, broiled	180	7.69	3.14	76
Top loin, broiled	176	7.99	3.20	65
Tenderloin, broiled	176	8.15	3.18	72
Bottom round, braised	191	8.47	3.01	81
Chuck arm pot roast, braised	199	8.77	3.33	85
Pork (lean only)				
Tenderloin, roasted	141	4.09	1.41	79
Ham, boneless, water added, extra lean (approximately 5% fat)	111	4.23	1.38	39
Ham, cured, center slice	165	7.08	2.37	(not available)
Center loin chop, broiled	196	8.91	3.07	83
Poultry (roasted)				
Turkey, light meat, without skin	131	2.48	.79	59
Chicken breast, meat only	140	3	.86	72
Chicken drumstick, meat only	146	4.8	1.26	79
Chicken breast, meat and skin	167	6.6	1.86	71
Chicken drumstick, meat and skin	184	9.47	2.59	77

Figures for 3-ounce cooked servings, with all visible fat removed and prepared with no added fat.
SOURCE: U.S. Dept. of Agriculture Handbooks No. 8-5, 8-10, and 8-13.

has figured all the food options up to 19 grams of fat and 620 calories per serving in Table 13.2. You won't be carrying this book to the store with you, so I suggest you make a copy of this table to put in your purse or wallet for easy reference.

A lot of busy working people eat microwave dinners several times a week. Most of these dinners are about 300 to 400 calories, but many are loaded with fat. Start checking them with this table. For instance, if you bought a 300-calorie microwave dinner with 14 grams of fat, it would have 42 percent fat calories. Try to buy a 300-calorie microwave dinner with no more than 10 fat grams (30 percent fat) and preferably closer to 7 (21 percent fat).

Can You Trust the Milkman?

When you reach into the dairy case for the "2 percent low-fat milk," are you buying it because you want to cut down on your fat intake, and does "2 percent" imply to you that 98 percent of the fat is removed? I have asked at least a thousand people these questions, and nine out of ten answer yes to both. You don't suppose the wholesome, squeaky-clean dairy industry would play labeling games with us, do you? I'll bet you a Holstein cow they would.

What if the milk carton read "only 3.3 percent fat"? Wouldn't you also assume that 96.7 percent of the fat had been removed? Wrong! That's Elsie's full load of fat. Like the meat processors, the milk industry quotes fat as a percentage of weight instead of as a percentage of calories. You will see in Table 13.3 that 3.3 percent is all the fat there is in whole milk—by weight.

The USDA has established standards of identity for milk based on fat content as determined by liquid weight. It permits the dairy companies to label milk "low fat" with anywhere from a 0.50 percent content, which is indeed low fat, all the way up to 2.00 percent—which isn't low fat by a country mile. Whole milk contains at least 3.25 percent fat.

How does all this shake out with fat as a percentage of calories? In the fat column in Table 13.3, you will see that 2 percent milk has 4.7 and whole milk 8.2 fat grams. A nutrition label reveals that the 2 percent milk rounds the 4.7 up to 5 grams and the whole milk 8.2 down to 8. The USDA permits rounding fractions to the nearest number. So what is prominently displayed on the front of

TABLE 13.2.

Fat as a percentage of total calories

	GRAMS OF FAT																		
	1	2	3	4	5	6	7	8	9	10	11	12	13	14	15	16	17	18	19
150	.06	.12	.18	.24	.30	.36	.42	.48	.54	.60	.66	.72	.78	.84	.90	.96			
160	.05	.11	.16	.22	.28	.33	.39	.45	.50	.56	.61	.67	.73	.78	.84	.90	.95		
170	.05	.10	.15	.21	.26	.31	.37	.42	.47	.52	.58	.63	.68	.74	.79	.84	.90	.95	
180	.05	.10	.15	.20	.25	.30	.35	.40	.45	.50	.55	.60	.65	.70	.75	.80	.85	.90	.95
190	.04	.09	.14	.18	.23	.28	.33	.37	.42	.47	.52	.56	.61	.66	.71	.75	.80	.85	.90
200	.04	.09	.13	.18	.22	.27	.31	.36	.40	.45	.49	.54	.58	.63	.67	.72	.76	.81	.85
210	.04	.08	.12	.17	.21	.25	.30	.34	.38	.42	.47	.51	.55	.60	.64	.68	.72	.77	.81
220	.04	.08	.12	.16	.20	.24	.28	.32	.36	.40	.45	.49	.53	.57	.61	.65	.69	.73	.77
230	.03	.07	.11	.15	.19	.23	.27	.31	.35	.39	.43	.46	.50	.54	.58	.62	.66	.70	.74
240	.03	.07	.11	.15	.18	.22	.26	.30	.33	.37	.41	.45	.48	.52	.56	.60	.63	.67	.71
250	.03	.17	.10	.14	.18	.21	.25	.28	.32	.36	.39	.43	.46	.50	.54	.57	.61	.64	.68
260	.03	.06	.10	.13	.17	.20	.24	.27	.31	.34	.38	.41	.45	.48	.51	.55	.58	.62	.65
270	.03	.06	.10	.13	.16	.20	.23	.26	.30	.33	.36	.40	.43	.46	.50	.53	.56	.60	.63
280	.03	.06	.09	.12	.16	.19	.22	.25	.28	.32	.35	.38	.41	.45	.48	.51	.54	.57	.61
290	.03	.06	.09	.12	.15	.18	.21	.24	.27	.31	.34	.37	.40	.43	.46	.49	.52	.55	.58
300	.03	.06	.09	.12	.15	.18	.21	.24	.27	.30	.33	.36	.39	.42	.45	.48	.51	.54	.57
310	.02	.05	.08	.11	.14	.17	.20	.23	.26	.29	.31	.34	.37	.40	.43	.46	.49	.52	.55
320	.02	.05	.08	.11	.14	.16	.19	.22	.25	.28	.30	.33	.36	.39	.42	.45	.47	.50	.53
330	.02	.05	.08	.10	.13	.16	.19	.21	.24	.27	.30	.32	.35	.38	.40	.43	.46	.49	.51
340	.02	.05	.07	.10	.13	.15	.18	.21	.23	.26	.29	.31	.34	.37	.39	.42	.45	.47	.50
350	.02	.05	.07	.10	.12	.15	.18	.20	.23	.25	.28	.30	.33	.36	.38	.41	.43	.46	.48
360	.02	.05	.07	.10	.12	.15	.17	.20	.22	.25	.27	.30	.32	.35	.37	.40	.42	.45	.47
370	.02	.04	.07	.09	.12	.14	.17	.19	.21	.24	.26	.29	.31	.34	.36	.38	.41	.43	.46
380	.02	.04	.07	.09	.11	.14	.16	.18	.21	.23	.26	.28	.30	.33	.35	.37	.40	.42	.45
390	.02	.04	.06	.09	.11	.13	.16	.18	.20	.23	.25	.27	.30	.32	.34	.36	.39	.41	.43
400	.02	.04	.06	.09	.11	.13	.15	.18	.20	.22	.24	.27	.29	.31	.33	.36	.38	.40	.42
410	.02	.04	.06	.08	.10	.13	.15	.17	.19	.21	.24	.26	.28	.30	.32	.35	.37	.39	.41
420	.02	.04	.06	.08	.10	.12	.15	.17	.19	.21	.23	.25	.27	.30	.32	.34	.36	.38	.40
430	.02	.04	.06	.08	.10	.12	.14	.16	.18	.20	.23	.25	.27	.29	.31	.33	.35	.37	.39
440	.02	.04	.06	.08	.10	.12	.14	.16	.18	.20	.22	.24	.26	.28	.30	.32	.34	.36	.38
450	.02	.04	.06	.08	.10	.12	.14	.16	.18	.20	.22	.24	.26	.28	.30	.32	.34	.36	.38
460	.01	.03	.05	.07	.09	.11	.13	.15	.17	.19	.21	.23	.25	.27	.29	.31	.33	.35	.37
470	.01	.03	.05	.07	.09	.11	.13	.15	.17	.19	.21	.22	.24	.26	.28	.30	.32	.34	.36
480	.01	.03	.05	.07	.09	.11	.13	.15	.16	.18	.20	.22	.24	.26	.28	.30	.31	.33	.35
490	.01	.03	.05	.07	.09	.11	.12	.14	.16	.18	.20	.22	.23	.25	.27	.29	.31	.33	.34
500	.01	.03	.05	.07	.09	.10	.12	.14	.16	.18	.19	.21	.23	.25	.27	.28	.30	.32	.34
510	.01	.03	.05	.07	.08	.10	.12	.14	.15	.17	.19	.21	.22	.24	.26	.28	.30	.31	.33
520	.01	.03	.05	.06	.08	.10	.12	.13	.15	.17	.19	.20	.22	.24	.25	.27	.29	.31	.32
530	.01	.03	.05	.06	.08	.10	.11	.13	.15	.16	.18	.20	.22	.23	.25	.27	.28	.30	.32
540	.01	.03	.05	.06	.08	.10	.11	.13	.15	.16	.18	.20	.21	.23	.25	.26	.28	.30	.31
550	.01	.03	.04	.06	.08	.09	.11	.13	.14	.16	.18	.19	.21	.22	.24	.26	.27	.29	.31
560	.01	.03	.04	.06	.08	.09	.11	.12	.14	.16	.17	.19	.20	.22	.24	.25	.27	.28	.30
570	.01	.03	.04	.06	.07	.09	.11	.12	.14	.15	.17	.18	.20	.22	.23	.25	.26	.28	.30
580	.01	.03	.04	.06	.07	.09	.10	.12	.13	.15	.17	.18	.20	.21	.23	.24	.26	.27	.29
590	.01	.03	.04	.06	.07	.09	.10	.12	.13	.15	.16	.18	.19	.21	.22	.24	.25	.27	.28
600	.01	.03	.04	.06	.07	.09	.10	.12	.13	.15	.16	.18	.19	.21	.22	.24	.25	.27	.28
610	.01	.02	.04	.05	.07	.08	.10	.11	.13	.14	.16	.17	.19	.20	.22	.23	.25	.26	.28
620	.01	.02	.04	.05	.07	.08	.10	.11	.13	.14	.15	.17	.18	.20	.21	.23	.24	.26	.27

(Row labels at left, reading vertically: C A L O R I E S)

TABLE 13.3.

TYPE OF MILK	CALORIES (per cup)	FAT (grams)	CALCIUM (milligrams)
Skim milk	86	0.4	302
Buttermilk, cultured	99	2.2	285
1% milk	102	2.6	300
2% milk	121	4.7	297
Whole milk, 3.3% fat	150	8.2	291
Chocolate milk, 2% fat	179	5.0	284
Chocolate milk, whole	208	8.5	280

SOURCE: Agriculture Handbook No. 8-1, USDA *Composition of Foods, Dairy and Egg Products*

the carton as "low fat" is actually five eighths of the total. When you have more than half of something, it doesn't qualify as "low" to me.

I drink very little milk, but I use a lot of it on cereal and in my hot tea. Skim milk has not only the fewest calories and least fat, but also, as shown on the chart, the highest calcium—a winning combination. If you are drinking 2 percent or whole milk, skim may seem thin and lacking in taste at first. If it does, mix it with 2 percent, and over time you can train your taste buds to like skim milk.

Cutting fat from your diet means reducing cheese—all kinds—to practically nothing. I confess that if there was one food I could have in unlimited amounts, I would want it to be cheese. Melted on various foods, added to a sandwich, or simply a wedge with some crackers, cheese hits my dietary hot button. Unfortunately, fat as a percentage of calories in a serving of cheese ranges from 60 to 85 percent. It is also mostly saturated fat, which is also a negative for cholesterol.

As you can tell by now, buying any kind of processed food involves a high risk of ending up with hidden fat that you didn't want. Ignore all the big, eye-catching numbers and phrases on the front of the package. Go right to the nutrition label and check the portion size and number of calories. Look for the fat grams per serving and compute the percentage of fat calories that the product has per serving. If it is over 30 percent, you should think hard about whether to buy it.

TRAINING THE TASTE BUDS

Eating smart is a process of reeducation. We all have taste preferences, and the daily decision-making process about what we will and won't eat is played out on the tops of our tongues by our taste buds. We learned early in life that sweet is good, and that sweet coupled with fat (chocolate cake, for instance) is doubly good. Not only that; sweet and fat were often elevated by offering them as a reward. I can still remember my mother saying, "Eat your carrots or you won't get any butterscotch pie" (my favorite as a kid). Is there anyone who hasn't heard that kind of ultimatum?

Regardless of how old you are, most of your taste preferences for sweet, fat foods were established at an early age, and the same taste-learning process continues for children today. Unfortunately, because of junk foods and high-fat school lunches, childhood obesity is becoming a national problem. The September 6, 1990, issue of *USA Today* reported that the most frequently served foods at school lunches were hamburgers, french fries, salad, chocolate cupcakes, and 2 percent milk. This menu has 1,081 calories, "about 47 percent from fat." Outside school, pizza and highly sugared colas are the favorites of most teenagers. These young taste buds are getting hooked early on the sweet-fat connection. That preference will be difficult for them to shake as they reach middle age and their weight starts to pile up.

Reeducating yourself to enjoy foods that are less fat and less sweet is not something that you should do abruptly. Cutting out everything you like is what restrictive diets are all about. Ultimately they fail because the weight goal is reached by temporarily altering normal eating choices. Most people can psych themselves up and keep their taste buds under control for a while in order to lose a certain number of pounds. But part of that resolve comes from knowing that the diet is only temporary. Oprah Winfrey did just that. She lived on a 400-calorie liquid diet just long enough to fit into size-10 jeans. Then, slowly but surely, her taste buds drew her back to her favorite foods, such as "butter glistening mashed potatoes made with horseradish, and key lime pie," according to *People*.

What happened to Oprah has happened to me at least a half

dozen times. I sympathize with her and know what a helpless feeling it is to crave a certain food, almost like an alcoholic craves a drink or a heavy smoker needs a cigarette. But why is it that we don't crave broccoli or carrots, which are healthful and on which we could pig out and not get fat?

The question "Why is it so hard to cut the fat?" was addressed in the May 1990 issue of Weight Watchers *Women's Health and Fitness News*. In the article, Dr. Adam Drewnowski, associate professor in the Human Nutrition Program at the University of Michigan School of Public Health in Ann Arbor, wrote: "There may be something to the idea that cravings and preferences for rich desserts are mediated by the same mechanism as drug addiction. . . . What people actually seem to crave is mixtures of fat and sugar, such as those found in ice cream, chocolate, candy, and chocolate chip cookies." He added that this may be because food preferences seem to be tied to the brain's opiate peptide system, which produces pleasure-enhancing molecules, such as endorphins, that have biochemical effects similar to those of opiate drugs. So sweet, fat cravings are not merely the result of weak willpower.

Studies show that the opiate-blocking drug naloxone hydrochloride, which is used to treat drug overdoses, blocks cravings for chocolate bars and cream-filled cookies in some people, according to Dr. Drewnowski. However, "the drug cannot be used for dieters because it must be given intravenously and is quickly cleared from the body." Studies conducted by Dr. Drewnowski and others at the University of Michigan found that overweight women prefer foods that are rich in fat and relatively low in sugar. "The fatter people were, the more they liked fat in their diet." This is a deadly cycle.

In the same article, Dr. Barbara J. Rolls, associate professor of psychiatry at Johns Hopkins Medical School, stated: "It's clear now that dietary fat is the key to body weight reduction." Dr. Rolls has done research to see whether altering the fat content of the diet during part of the day affects total calorie intake. She discovered that if the reduction in fat is small, people tend to eat other foods to compensate for the loss of fat calories, but that they don't eat *more* fat. Other studies have shown that, if people eat several reduced-fat foods throughout the day, their intake of both fat and calories drops. Obviously, then, the object is to *reduce* fat in the diet, not try to eliminate it.

The battle we all face is to reduce fat intake while satisfying our taste buds. Most flavor preferences are learned (usually culturally), but a couple are inborn. For instance, babies prefer sweet flavors from birth, and bitterness is universally disliked from birth. Bitter, though, can become an acquired taste, such as for black coffee or quinine water. If you make a concerted effort to reeducate your taste buds to like certain foods and liquids that are good for you, you will eat and drink them more often. It should be a gradual process, however.

In the Western industrialized countries, and in particular the United States, meat and dairy products are introduced into our diets early, and our taste buds get hooked on them. In other countries, taste preferences develop for totally different foods. China, for instance, does not have a dairy industry, so milk and butter are rare. In fact, the Chinese call butter "cow oil" and consider its taste repugnant. The eating habits we learn as young children create an "indelible blueprint for adult behavior patterns," according to Kathy Duran.

People who want to control their weight and eat nutritiously must also retrain their minds. Meat and dairy products should be deemphasized in favor of whole grains, vegetables, and fruits. We must unlearn some of our early beliefs about why we need to eat a lot of meat protein and to ingest a lot of dairy products for calcium. There are other, more healthful ways to get adequate protein and calcium.

Today's typical diet in Western industrialized countries is much higher in animal fat and protein than we need or should have, and this raises the risks of cancer, heart disease, obesity, diabetes, and osteoporosis. Studies show that the average American eats about twice as much protein as needed. There has been an overemphasis on protein (i.e., meat), and in my view the USDA has designed its guidelines for the benefit of the meat and dairy producers.

THE PREHISTORIC DIET

In *The Paleolithic Prescription*, Dr. S. Boyd Eaton, Marjorie Shostak, and Dr. Melvin Konner analyze the dietary intake and lifestyles of our ancestors of 40,000 years ago, when the human species were hunter-gatherers. This was before the advent of agriculture and domesticated animals. A persuasive case is made that we should blend the best dietary and exercise features from the past with the best from the present. The authors point out that between 1910 and 1976 consumption of fats in the United States increased by about 25 percent, so that today fat makes up about 42 percent on average of the calories we consume each day. "This level of fat consumption is unprecedented in human evolutionary experience and results in diseases that kill us, but that are uncommon in countries where fat represents a much smaller portion of the diet."

The diet in rural Japan is cited. Only 10 to 12 percent of the daily calories come from fat, and the prevalence of coronary heart disease among rural Japanese is just a fraction of ours. Recent studies show, however, that when Japanese move to Western industrialized countries and increase their fat intake, they also evidence an increase in heart disease.

It is difficult for us to realize that the 10,000 years since agriculture and domesticated animals came on the scene is only an instant in terms of our total evolutionary development. It took millions of years to develop our upright bipedal locomotion system. Our physical-activity requirements and dietary needs were being developed at the same time. Now, in just a few years by evolutionary standards, we have nearly eliminated physical activity and drastically altered the composition and quantity of food that we eat. This has played havoc with the way we accumulate and store fat. The authors of *The Paleolithic Prescription* point out that the fat-storage pattern of free-living mammals other than humans is fairly uniform. For instance, have you ever noticed that a herd of zebras or wildebeests on the plains of Africa all look as if they weigh about the same? The deer and coyotes that frequently pass through my rural acreage are also uniform in size. As the authors state, "The range of body composition in wild animal species is relatively narrow."

As we human animals got smarter, we learned how to produce a year-round supply of food. The hunter-gatherer life of our prehistoric ancestors became obsolete, and as a result our body composition changed from what was once a moderately uniform range to an extreme one. Now human body-fat composition can vary between 2 and 60 percent of our total weight, according to Eaton, Shostak, and Konner. Unlike wild animals, humans similar in age, height, and sex differ widely in the amount of fat they carry. The unlimited amount of high-density fat calories available in most Western countries, with so little physical effort needed to obtain them, makes excess fat an inevitable consequence. A few centuries ago, only the wealthy were fat, but now that condition has reversed. Obesity is a hallmark of the lower socioeconomic level, while the educated and well-to-do have the knowledge and desire to maintain a healthier weight range. As *The Paleolithic Prescription* points out, "This transfer of obesity to the poor is occurring at the same time as obesity's harmful health effects are becoming well documented."

Stone Age people were lean, strong, aerobically fit, and almost totally free from the chronic diseases that cause 75 percent of all deaths in the United States today. The authors state: "Our genetic make-up—designed over millions of years and largely unchanged in the last ten thousand—has become sharply discordant with life today; drastic changes in human nutrition and exercise patterns have promoted cancer, heart disease, diabetes, hypertension, obesity, and even tooth decay." Clearly, being overfed and underexercised contributes to poor health and lessened longevity. If you are fat, health is the primary and maybe the *only* reason you should lose weight, because fat culls the human herd quietly and quickly. Obituaries never list fat as the cause of death, but we now know that it produces a friendly environment for adult diabetes, some cancers, heart disease, and hypertension. Such diseases are listed on the official death record, but excess fat is the silent, lethal accomplice.

A LITTLE KNOWLEDGE ELIMINATES A LOT OF FAT

With the amount of processed, fast, and snack food we all consume, it is impossible to win the dietary fat game without learning some of the rules. Unfortunately, the rules keep changing, so the learning process should never end. Most people, though, are nutritional illiterates; some because they don't care about what they eat and how it may affect their health, others because they simply don't know where to get up-to-date, accurate information about nutrition.

I was one of these until eight years ago, when I realized I must control my cholesterol or risk heart problems. It was remarkable how my life changed once I became curious about exercise and nutrition. The more I learned, the more control I had over my weight and fitness. The most interesting aspect of learning the low-fat, high–complex carbohydrate way of eating is that I do not eat a single thing I do not like. What *has* changed is that I like many more foods and now eat a greater variety of them. I have found that the more I read and understand about the way my body functions and the fuel it needs, the easier it is to maintain proper weight and a healthy life-style. Here is my recommended reading list that will keep you up to date with reliable nutritional information. There are others that are good, but I consider these three newsletters the best:

University of California at Berkeley Wellness Letter
Subscription Department
P.O. Box 420148
Palm Coast, FL 32142

I have taken this letter for nine years and look forward to it every month. It is easy to read and covers nutrition, exercise, and all subjects related to wellness.

Tufts University Diet and Nutrition Letter
Subscription Department
P.O. Box 57857
Boulder, CO 80322-7857

This fine letter focuses mostly on diet and nutrition. It is also easy to read and understand. I have quoted from it in this chapter and consider it a reliable source.

Mayo Clinic Health Letter
Subscription Department
Rochester, MN 55903-9915

Published by the internationally famous Mayo Clinic, this letter will keep you informed about the many aspects of proper nutrition and health.

Don't be intimidated by health and nutrition letters from universities or places like the Mayo Clinic. They are written so that we can readily understand them.

Prevention magazine combines the best of exercise with the best of nutrition, and it has been a proponent of exercise walking and low-fat eating for many years. It has articles by chefs on how to cook low-fat meals, nutritional information, and inspirational stories about people who have won their fat battle. You can buy

Prevention at newsstands or subscribe to it by writing Customer Communications, Rodale Press, 33 East Minor Street, Emmaus, PA 18098.

There is a book on nutrition that I urge everyone to read. It is *Jane Brody's Good Food Book: Living the High-Carbohydrate Way*. Jane Brody is the personal health columnist of *The New York Times*, and it was her first best-seller, *Nutrition*, that got me interested ten years ago in what I was pumping through my digestive system. It was then that I realized I was nutritionally illiterate.

One other source of information (and perhaps inspiration) is Weight Watchers. This is the oldest weight-loss organization in the country. Weight Watchers is fairly inexpensive for an individual, and there are even units within companies. My daughter, Molly, a senior design artist at Hallmark in Kansas City who has a stubbornly slow metabolism, regularly attends the Weight Watchers group that meets there. Weekly encouragement helps her to stay on track. By joining Weight Watchers you will get current nutritional information and counseling. More important, you will meet and talk with others who are also struggling with their weight. You will probably find that there are some who are worse off than you. Weight Watchers will help you replace self-pity with determination, and then you will be on your way.

RANDOM TIPS ON FIGHTING FAT

Over the past eight years I have learned a number of things that help make the fat fight a breeze. Here are ten ideas that work for me and may help you.

GRAZING: I picked this idea up in *Jane Brody's Good Food Book*. (She didn't call it grazing, but the principle is the same.) Eat five or six small, low-fat meals through the day instead of two or three big ones, of which the largest is usually the evening meal. Our prehistoric ancestors were grazers; they were constantly moving about trying to find food. Only in modern times do we sit down at prescribed times to eat. Drink a full glass of water before each snack, and you will rarely be hungry. (This also helps you get your necessary water intake.) Sometimes I eat three bowls of cereal in the course of a day, with fresh fruit, skim milk, and NutraSweet. It drives Carol nuts, but I think cereal and fruit make a great low-fat dessert!

YOGURT-CEREAL LUNCH: My favorite lunch is Kellogg's Shredded Wheat Squares (blueberry, raisin, or apple cinnamon) in a bowl with Weight Watchers 90-calorie no-fat fruit yogurt and a tablespoon of Grape-Nuts. Stir this up, and you'll have a delicious lunch. You will be stuffed but will have taken in only a couple of hundred calories and *no* fat calories. When they are available, add fresh strawberries, blueberries, or raspberries.

FORGET THE BUTTER: I have not had butter or margarine on bread or toast in five years. At breakfast I usually top a piece of Carol's toasted homemade seven-grain bread with strawberry preserves. Learn to leave the butter or margarine off. Preserves or jelly only has about 18 calories a teaspoon and no fat. Your taste buds won't know the difference. Honey, jelly, preserves, and apple butter are great substitutes for butter or margarine and save a lot of fat intake. A few calories of sugar are a better trade-off than a lot of calories of fat.

PRETZELS OVER POTATO CHIPS: When you feel the craving for something crunchy and salty, get pretzels. Read the label, however, because some are lower in fat and have less sodium than others. Compared with potato chips or peanuts, pretzels are an excellent light snack.

NEW POTATOES: We all have a need for crunchy food from time to time. That's why liquid diets soon become a problem. New potatoes are small red- or tan-skinned potatoes. Clean three or four that are not much bigger than oversized English walnuts and eat them raw, as you would an apple, skin and all. They are crunchy, delicious, and about as nutritious as anything you can eat. If you don't have a sodium problem, sprinkle a little salt on them. Four small potatoes have less than 100 calories and no fat calories. Don't knock it if you haven't tried it.

PORTION CONTROL: I win a lot of bets with Carol on what portion size equals 4 or 5 ounces of a given food. We haul out our kitchen scale, which weighs in grams and ounces, and weigh a portion. She generally has prepared enough to feed a lumberjack in each portion, so we cut it down. Most people underestimate portion sizes and end up eating more than they realize. A small kitchen scale is a good investment. It will help you train your eye to judge portions.

THE TWO-BITE DESSERT: At the end of a low-fat meal, sometimes the desire for a sweet, fat dessert becomes irresistible. If you turn it down, you'll still be thinking about it at 3:00 A.M. Here's my solution. At a restaurant, Carol and I mutually agree on a dessert, order one with two forks, and limit ourselves to two normal bites. I eat mine very slowly and keep it on my tongue as long as possible, letting it dissolve like a piece of hard candy. This gives my taste buds the sweet, fat fix they were screaming for. I have taken in only a small amount of fat calories, yet I have satisfied my craving. By eating only two bites, you also reinforce your discipline. Just as important, you feel a lot better than if you ate the whole dish and then wished you hadn't. How many times have you done that?

BLENDER GLOP: I have fun throwing food into a blender to see what combinations taste like. One of my favorites is a cup of crushed ice, a cup of orange juice, any Weight Watchers 90-calorie, no-fat fruit yogurt, a banana, fresh strawberries if available, and a packet of NutraSweet. Run the blender for a minute or until everything is thoroughly combined. If it is too thick to pour easily, add a little water or more ice and blend again. Pour the result over ice cubes in a big glass and grate nutmeg on top. This is tastier than a milk shake and very filling without any fat calories.

LOW FAT AT 30,000 FEET: I meet many business executives at the Cooper Wellness Program who say one of their biggest problems is the number of airline meals they have to eat because of their heavy travel schedules. Airline meals are notoriously loaded with fat calories. Always have your travel agent order the "low-cholesterol meal" for you when your reservation is made, or order it yourself if you make your own reservations. Do this even if you don't have a cholesterol problem. You will get a low-fat meal such as fresh fruit, broiled skinless chicken breast, whole wheat bun, diet margarine, a vegetable, and rice. As a rule, it is pretty tasty. Generally someone sitting next to me eating the regular airline goo enviously asks how I got such a good meal. Even if it is only a snack flight, you will probably get a turkey breast sandwich instead of ham and cheese.

DON'T SKIP BREAKFAST: More people skip breakfast than any other meal, yet it is the most important one of all. There's an old saying: "Eat breakfast like a king or queen, eat lunch like a prince or princess, and eat dinner like a pauper." Many dieters think a quick cup of coffee in the morning without breakfast will help reduce their calorie intake. At the end of the day, however, most of them have consumed more calories than if they had started their day with a nutritious breakfast. Jane Brody makes an interesting case for breakfast in her *Good Food Book*, citing a study from Johns Hopkins University of people in their 80s and 90s. Most of them had always eaten a large breakfast. A low-fat, high-energy breakfast should start everyone's day. If you are going to lighten up on calories, do it at the evening meal.

For a 64-year-old retired businessman to be passing on tips to you about nutrition and weight control is proof positive that you really can teach an old dog new tricks. Until eight years ago, I wouldn't even try a lot of fruits and vegetables. Everything I ate had to be sweet, fat, or both. Now nothing goes in my mouth unless I know that it is healthful, and low in fat and cholesterol. This old dog, who wants to live to be a lot older, has changed his eating pattern from gluttonous gratification to smart eating. Give it a chance. Eating smart works for me, and it will for you too. But don't forget your daily walk.

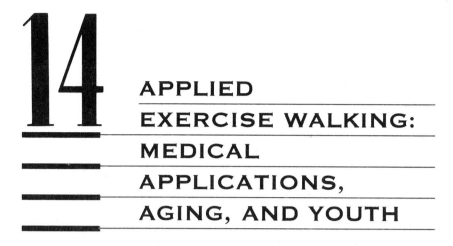

APPLIED
EXERCISE WALKING:
MEDICAL
APPLICATIONS,
AGING, AND YOUTH

In early 1985, at a roundtable discussion on the merits of exercise by medical doctors and exercise physiologists, Robert F. DeBusk, M.D., associate professor of medicine and director of the Cardiac Rehabilitation Program for the Stanford (California) University School of Medicine, stated in *The Physician and Sportsmedicine* that when physicians recommend exercise "they gain nothing and lose a lot when patients come back with shin splints and other orthopedic nuisances." He added, "Most people are advised to exercise at levels that are excessive."

Dr. DeBusk's reference to "shin splints and other orthopedic nuisances" is indicative of the exercises (jogging, running, and high-impact aerobics) that were in vogue in early 1985. His comment is well taken. Why prescribe a remedy that will only compound the ailment? Other doctors, particularly orthopedic doctors, had been warning about these problems as far back as 1979. Also in vogue in the go-go eighties was the idea that exercise must be highly intensive to be effective, and Dr. DeBusk appropriately was urging caution.

At the time this roundtable was held, the walking movement was silently gathering momentum. It obviously wasn't the culprit for shinsplints because, as late as September 1984, the CDC Workshop reported, "Empirical data about the risk of walking, the most common activity, are absent." Walking is now well entrenched as the nation's number-one exercise, and concerns about its orthopedic problems are almost nonexistent. In addition, its intensity levels are easily regulated, and a substantial effort is required for the average person to walk at an "excessive level."

MEDICAL APPLICATIONS

Although this book is primarily focused on walking for fitness and weight control, there are a number of diseases and rehabilitative procedures—such as cardiac rehabilitation, hypertension, stroke, adult diabetes, arthritis, and loss of functional mobility from aging—that respond best when exercise is part of the treatment. Those of you who have the normal function of your walking gait and any of the foregoing problems will find that walking is the ideal exercise to aid in your treatment.

My friend Neil F. Gordon, M.D., Ph.D., M.P.H., who is director of exercise physiology at the Institute for Aerobics Research and director of the Aerobics Center Cardiac Rehabilitation Program, has kindly provided some of the medical counsel about the previously mentioned diseases for this chapter. He advises that all this exercise information should be implemented only in consultation with your physician.

Cardiac Rehabilitation

Since the early 1980s, predischarge (before going home from the hospital) exercise testing has been a recognized cardiac diagnostic tool. This permits the patient to stress his heart in a controlled environment with a doctor and nurse in attendance. Dr. Gordon says, "Most experts now believe that these exercise test results can tell a physician more about a patient's risk for future cardiac complications than the results of any other single procedure." A favorable test result also has important psychological effects, not only for patients but for spouses and loved ones, for it helps to smooth the transition back to a normal life.

Once you have been tested and sent home, the process of cardiac rehabilitation and the many variables that can affect it are quite involved. The more you know about "cardiac rehab," the better you will feel, physically and mentally. Dr. Gordon and Dr. Larry W. Gibbons, the Cooper Clinic's medical director, have written a book titled *The Cooper Clinic Cardiac Rehabilitation Program.* It is directed to the general reader and touches on every aspect of the subject. It covers many details about recuperation and rehabilitation that may not come up in the normal doctor-patient exchange.

Obviously exercise is a critical component of cardiac rehabilitation, and Drs. Gordon and Gibbons have examined all the pros and cons of the exercise choices, much as I did in Chapter 7. They conclude: "Most experts, including ourselves, consider walking the most appropriate aerobic activity for coronary artery disease patients." One of the reasons it is appropriate is that walking intensity is easy to control, so even those in the high-risk category can walk and get the desired conditioning effect. They cite another reason: "It is one of the least likely to cause musculoskeletal problems." I have been preaching about this for a dozen chapters.

Many patients have spectacular recoveries from heart attacks or heart surgery and became aggressive exercisers because they want to develop a maximum level of cardiovascular fitness. All too often these exercisers have been advised to use walking for their initial rehabilitation but to seek higher exercise intensity with running, cycling, or some other exercise. Aerobic walking as described in Chapter 6 will give anyone the fitness of a runner without risk of injury. In addition, heart patients will get from walking the specificity-of-training effect that helps them function better in their daily life. As Dr. Gordon said to me, "Anyone can derive *all* of their health and fitness needs from a walking program."

Hypertension

Hypertension (high blood pressure) is the most common cardio-vascular disease, affecting about 58 million Americans, with more than half having some degree of heart involvement. More than 60,000 deaths a year are attributable to hypertension and hypertensive heart disease. According to Dr. Gordon, "Epidemiological studies suggest that regular participation in physical activity may be beneficial in preventing hypertension." There is reason to believe that aerobic exercise training may reduce the mortality rate in hypertensive patients.

Aerobic exercise training can be effective in controlling mild hypertension without medication in some cases, or it may be used in conjunction with medication. Dr. Gordon recommends an aerobic intensity of 60 to 85 percent of the maximal heart rate. He says that exercise duration and frequency should be regulated so that about 1,000 to 2,000 calories a week are expended. Many people who engage in this level of exercise are ultimately able to discontinue high-blood-pressure medication. Walking is the ideal exercise to produce these physiological results.

Stroke

It is not commonly known, but stroke is the third leading cause of death in the United States, after heart disease and all types of cancer combined. A stroke is a potentially fatal cutoff of the blood supply to part of the brain. When the blood supply to any part of the brain is reduced, the oxygen-starved cells in that area stop functioning properly. For those who survive a stroke and whose rehabilitation program has brought them to a stage at which only a slight to moderate disability remains, a regular exercise program will help increase functional capacity and lessen the chance of having another stroke.

Dr. Gordon warns: "Stroke is a *recurrent* disease, and if you've had one stroke you are five times more likely to have others. To put it another way, of the 62 percent of people who survive a stroke, about one quarter can expect to have a second stroke unless they do something to prevent it." This is one of the primary reasons he believes that you should start exercising once your formal stroke rehabilitation program is over—that is, if you can. Not every stroke survivor recovers enough to be able to exercise regularly.

In his book *Stroke: Exercising Your Options*, Dr. Gordon writes: "Moderate exertion several days a week is likely to greatly reduce the chances that you'll develop a second stroke or die prematurely from other various potentially chronic diseases." Just as important, exercise will help reduce your disability. Even though you may have to walk with a slight limp caused by irreversible neurologic impairment, you may be able to increase the distance you can walk, which reduces your degree of disability. If you are a stroke survivor who is lucky enough still to have a good, functioning walking gait, use it for all it's worth. It can be your ticket to a longer, healthier life.

Diabetes

Diabetes is a complicated disease that affects some 10 million Americans. There are several types that respond to diet, exercise, and insulin, but Dr. Gordon advises that the largest numbers of people are afflicted with non-insulin-dependent diabetes mellitus (Type II). This is commonly called adult-onset diabetes because it is usually, though not always, discovered after the age of 30. For those with Type II diabetes, Dr. Gordon believes exercise should be a mainstay of the effort to control blood glucose. He says, "On the priority list, it comes right after eating correctly."

One of the reasons people develop Type II diabetes is that their cells have grown resistant or insensitive to the insulin circulating in the blood. According to Dr. Gordon, exercise improves insulin sensitivity. Weight loss also increases insulin sensitivity by lowering the liver's glucose production, which in turn improves blood-glucose control. "Getting weight down into the ideal range is often the only treatment that Type II diabetic patients need to normalize their blood-glucose levels," Dr. Gordon writes.

As pointed out in Chapter 12, exercise walking is the most effective, sustainable exercise for weight control, and it would be particularly effective for someone with Type II diabetes. Someone with diabetes should consult their doctor before embarking on an exercise program, however. Dr. Gordon cautions that for a diabetic a treadmill stress test should be conducted because of a condition known as silent heart disease. Diabetics suffer nerve damage and often lose the ability to feel pain. They are also more prone to heart attacks than non-diabetics. A treadmill test will help disclose heart disease in a diabetic who might not feel the chest pain associated with it.

A diabetic should be extra cautious about getting blisters from shoes or socks. His or her healing process is not good, so extra preventive care should be taken to avoid blisters. A good walking program in consultation with your doctor will put you in charge of your weight, elevate your energy level, and give you the self-confidence you need to control your diabetes.

In addition to the foregoing, exercise walking will make you fit, which is a major plus for a diabetic. Figure 14.1 shows that fit men with high blood glucose and/or diabetes had about the same death rate as unfit men with normal blood-glucose levels. Fit men with

FIGURE 14.1

Study involving 8,118 male Cooper Clinic patients over an eight-year period

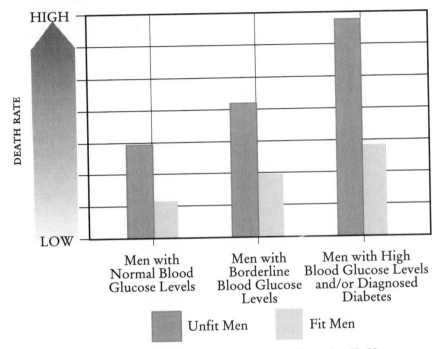

SOURCE: Neil F. Gordon, *Diabetes: Exercising Your Options*. Champaign, IL: Human Kinetics, in press.

borderline blood glucose actually did better than the unfit men with normal levels.

Few diseases are as responsive to a lifetime exercise program as Type II adult-onset diabetes, and few exercises are as sustainable for a lifetime as exercise walking. If you are one of the unfortunate people with Type II diabetes, take charge of your life in a forceful, positive way and start walking.

Arthritis

"I can buy you some time" was the candid comment from the orthopedic surgeon who performed a 2½-hour arthroscopic debridement on my right knee on January 13, 1987. It was the third operation on the knee since 1973, and the advanced osteoarthritis was evident in the X rays even to my untrained eye. Someday, as the doctor implied, I may have to have an artificial knee, but five years after the operation I am still walking every day (though some days better than others), and I believe it is the constant exercise that is prolonging the time until my day of reckoning.

Because of my advancing age and the tenuous state of my arthritic knee, I was particularly interested in Dr. Gordon's book *Arthritis: Exercising Your Options*. According to it, almost half of all Americans 65 years or older have some debilitating arthritic condition. Even about 28 percent of Americans between 45 and 64 years old have some form of arthritis. The word *arthritis* is derived from two Greek words, *arthron* (means "joint") and *itis* (means "inflammation"). Literally, it means "inflammation of the joint," and those of us who have it can certainly attest to this.

Osteoarthritis has the distinction of being the oldest and most prevalent chronic disease known to humankind, according to Dr. Gordon. Damage is limited to the musculoskeletal system, usually in weight-bearing joints—feet, knees, hips, and spine. However, it also invades the digital joints of the fingers, hands, and toes. Until recently, experts thought osteoarthritis resulted from normal wear and tear on joints, but current thinking is that a variety of factors are responsible. Dr. Gordon writes: "Aging, repetitive impact on the body's weight-bearing joints, genetics, and some other as yet unknown biochemical processes are responsible for osteoarthritis."

For centuries rest was viewed as the only way to alleviate arthritis. Even gentle exercise was considered harmful. This has all changed, and for several decades doctors have been prescribing stretching exercises because they help to preserve joint function. Dr. Gordon points out that recent evidence indicates that aerobic exercise can aid in arthritis rehabilitation, "provided the exercise regimen is individually tailored for each patient and is coupled with appropriate rest."

The amount of "appropriate rest" creates a dilemma. Arthritis generally results in the greatest long-term disability of all chronic diseases, but Dr. Gordon believes that many physicians are still a bit too cautious and conservative in their exercise prescriptions. While rest helps reduce joint inflammation, excessive rest is deleterious. In only one week of immobilization, a muscle can lose about 30 percent of its bulk.

"Arthritis sufferers' main sources of physical discomfort are joint stiffness and pain," Dr. Gordon writes. "There is documented proof that appropriate exercise can help alleviate both." It is also true that inappropriate exercise worsens arthritis pain. This is especially true if the arthritis is currently active with inflammation.

As people age beyond 60, they tend to slow down, even if they don't have arthritis. Arthritis compounds the effects of inactivity and contributes to the wasting of muscles; weakness of muscles, ligaments, tendons, and bones; degeneration of joint cartilage; and "contractures," which reduce the range of a joint's mobility. Clearly there is more reason for someone who is arthritic to exercise than for someone who is not.

Obviously the level of an individual's arthritis determines what exercises are appropriate. Dr. Gordon says, "The preferred exercises are low-impact aerobics such as walking, cycling, and swimming." Your doctor's consultation is advised to determine if a weight-bearing exercise such as walking would be beneficial. People with advanced osteoarthritis would probably find more tolerable, sustainable exercise in the buoyancy of a swimming pool. In addition to the exercises mentioned, Dr. Gordon states: *"Daily range-of-motion exercises for the affected joints are absolutely essential"* (emphasis in original).

My personal case of osteoarthritis is still in a manageable state, but I don't baby myself. There are times I could decide not to walk, but by so doing I might be doing more overall damage to myself. Inflammation comes and goes. A little aspirin and a couple of days off now and then buy me another month or two of pain-free walking. Don't throw in the towel if you have arthritis. Inactivity and lack of exercise are your worst enemies. Pick an exercise you can tolerate in relation to your arthritic condition and go for it. If walking is tolerable, you will find it contributes hugely to your fitness, attitude, weight control, and sense of well-being.

WALKING AND AGING

How old is "old"? According to a survey in *Modern Maturity*, when asked to define *old age*, people under 30 said 63 was old; people 30 to 39 said 67 was old; people 40 to 49 said 70 was old; people 50 to 59 said 71 was old; people 60 to 64 said 73 was old; and people 65 plus said 75 was old. Notice that, as people age, they keep moving the goalposts back. I am 64, fit, trim, and healthy; 73 sure doesn't look old to me, because it's only nine years away!

Old age must be viewed from two perspectives. One is simply the chronology of years; the second, but more important, is the functional-activity level of the individual. At 64, I have a higher energy level and am actually in better physical condition than when I was 32, sedentary, and 52 pounds heavier. I see this same disparity in almost every one of my walking clinics. Highly active 70- and even some 80-year-olds outperform sedentary 50- and 60-year-olds. Although they may be older in years, their eyes are brighter, their step is quicker, their balance is better, their energy level is higher, and their outlook on life is more upbeat. What gives them this edge when they are 20 years older in age? Exercise!

I don't mean just any exercise; I mean walking, and lots of it. As people age, the range of exercises they can and should do narrows considerably. Most older people, especially women, can't tolerate a high-impact exercise like running. Exercise walking becomes the most obvious choice for the older population. More than any other activity, walking (because of the specificity principle) conditions the aging exerciser's primary gait of locomotion so that he or she can continue to function in normal, necessary activities. Inability simply to take care of minimal daily personal needs is a major problem of aging.

Many people in their 60s, 70s, and 80s who are sitting in wheelchairs in nursing homes have no specific ambulatory or orthopedic problems but have simply ceased to function. They have lost their ability to walk. Perhaps the term that describes this condition best is *progressive wasting of muscle tissue*. Dr. Steven Blair, director of epidemiology at the Institute for Aerobics Research, told me that he was discussing the aging population and its problems with Dr. Irwin Rosenberg, who used the term. Dr. Rosenberg is the director of the Human Nutrition Research Center on Aging at Tufts University.

Dr. Blair said that Dr. Rosenberg told him that this is a serious medical disorder and a national problem. Dr. Rosenberg believes that progressive wasting of muscle tissue is a condition requiring study and definition, and that ultimately it should be given a medical name. The well-known term *osteoporosis* evolved from this process. Drs. Blair and Rosenberg believe that many people can reverse the wasting-of-muscle-tissue problem by becoming active again. There is ample evidence to support their position.

The *University of California at Berkeley Wellness Letter* reported that many experts estimate that half the functional losses that set in between the ages of 30 and 70 are attributable to lack of exercise. When aging is accompanied by inactivity, it can result in declines on the following scales: "(1) Muscle fiber is lost at the rate of 3–5% a decade after age 30, leading to a 30% loss of muscle power by the age of 60; (2) By middle age, blood vessels typically narrow by 29%. Between the ages of 25 and 60, the circulation of blood from arms to legs slows down by as much as 60% and (3) The speed at which messages travel from the brain to the nerve endings decreases 10–15% by the age of 70." Although the foregoing occurs with inactivity and aging, regular exercise has been shown to inhibit, arrest, or even reverse such declines. It is time for you to take stock of your age and your exercise program (if you have one) to see if you are doing all that is necessary to help stall the aging process. If you are over 65 and aren't exercising, you are becoming a prime candidate for a nursing home.

The *Wellness Letter* reported that, if you were 65 in 1990, you have a 43 percent chance of living in a nursing home at some point. As people age and their inactivity increases, they reach what Dr. Blair calls a "functional disability threshold." They lose mobility to the extent that they don't have the physical capacity to take care of such simple personal needs as going to the grocery store. At this point nursing homes become the only alternative for most of them. Inactivity is a compounding, debilitating cycle, and within nursing homes people develop an inactivity threshold in which they are not even mobile enough to go to the bathroom or walk to the dining room.

Many of these people have simply lost their ability to walk. Probably more than half have what Dr. Rosenberg refers to as the progressive wasting of muscle tissue. This can be reversed if walking is reintroduced into their lives. Strangely, many will have to relearn this first and most significant activity they learned as a child. As Dr. Inman points out in *Human Walking*, walking is not a reflex action but a neural process and must be learned.

When learning to walk, children fall many times but get up and do it again. An 80-year-old who falls while relearning how to walk may never get up again. For many elderly people the fear of falling is one of the greatest terrors. The Associated Press reported that falls are the sixth leading cause of death in the elderly, and a fractured hip is among the most common and debilitating health problems that older people face.

David Oliver, head of rehabilitation, chronic, and long-term care services at the Heartland Health System in St. Joseph, Missouri, says, "The fear of falling in the elderly is immense. Their perception is: 'If I fall, I will break my hip. If I break my hip, I will go to the hospital. The next step is the nursing home, and the next stop is the funeral home. My whole life-style will change. I've seen it among my friends. If I break my hip, I'll never return home.'" Oliver believes this fear of falling may actually contribute to accidents, because as people reduce their activities their muscles become weaker and they lose coordination.

The more we do something, the better we are able to do it. The best solution to functional inactivity in the elderly is to encourage people to walk a lot in their earlier years so that they never stop.

As an exercise, the walking gait has been so poorly understood and underutilized that many nursing homes may not be equipped, or their staffs trained adequately, to teach the dysfunctional elderly how to walk again. The first concern is to eliminate the possibility of falls. All hallways should have handrails on both sides. For those who have regressed the most, a walking training area with double handrails should be available so that they can practice walking between the rails for physical safety and mental confidence. Eliminating the fear of falling is a major concern, second in importance only to eliminating falling itself.

Why do the elderly fall so much? Oliver says physical disabilities such as inner-ear problems that affect balance, fluctuating blood pressure, failing eyesight, the effects of strokes, anemia, and dementia are contributing factors. Perhaps the most overlooked reason, he believes, is too much medication, which can cause disorienting side effects when administered in different combinations. Certainly environmental factors such as slippery floors or uneven carpets also contribute to the problem. When all things are considered, however, if a properly structured walking program is put in place, many of the functionally disabled elderly can be taught to walk again safely. On a risk-reward basis, walking is still the most important exercise for them because it can restore their functional mobility.

While writing this book, I saw on TV some elderly men and women in a nursing home using exercise cycles. Most were hardly pedaling, so they probably weren't getting much real exercise.

Unfortunately, when they get off the exercise cycle they can't walk any better. Sitting and pedaling contributes nothing to balance and agility, nor does it condition walking muscles; only walking does that. The specificity principle should be the overriding guide in devising exercise for the elderly. How much pedaling does an 80-year-old need in order to function? By contrast, if all 80-year-olds could still walk well, a lot of nursing homes would be out of business.

Not only can 80-year-olds be retaught how to walk, but the results can be spectacular and they enjoy it. As this chapter is being written, David Oliver has kept me informed of an exercise program at the Heartland Health Facility. Seventeen people (15 women and 2 men) with an average age of 85 are doing something called Walk to Washington. The program starts at 11:00 A.M., and it has become the focal point of their day. In three months they have accumulated 170 miles, which is equivalent to walking from St. Joseph to Hannibal, Missouri. One of the women walkers is 101 years old.

Oliver says that most of the walkers, but especially several who are recovering from fractured hips, started out tentatively. Some walked looking down at their feet. The longest distance covered in a day by a walker is four city blocks, and the shortest is only 100 feet, but to every participant it is an accomplishment of which he or she is proud. The hospital staff reports that all of them have better appetites and better morale, are more animated, and sleep better. Even this small amount of mobility widens their horizons. Everything in life is relevant, right up to our last breath.

A health goal for anyone reading this book who is 60 or older is to maintain an activity level that can extend his or her ability to remain independent and mobile. Dr. Neil Gordon calls the loss of independent living "compressed morbidity," and Figure 14.2 explains this loss of functionality. For the aging population—and it includes me—walking combined with stretching and flexibility exercises constitutes the perfect exercise combination. Walking is gentle and its intensity is easily regulated to accommodate all levels of fitness. Unlike most other exercises, walking contributes directly to the all-important aspect of functional mobility.

After studying the compressed-morbidity chart in Figure 14.2, I have decided on the way I would like to go to the hereafter. If Dr. Gordon will move that bottom dot over to 100, when my time comes I want to *walk* down to the undertaker and expire on his doorstep. A tough old walker might as well save the pickup fee.

FIGURE 14.2
Compressed morbidity

This example shows theoretical curves for two individuals. The line labeled independent living indicates a threshold of function required for living independently. When a person's functional capability falls below this threshold, he or she must be institutionalized or receive custodial care. In this example, both people die at age ninety. The sedentary person had to be institutionalized for the last ten years of life, while the active person can live independently until near the end of life.

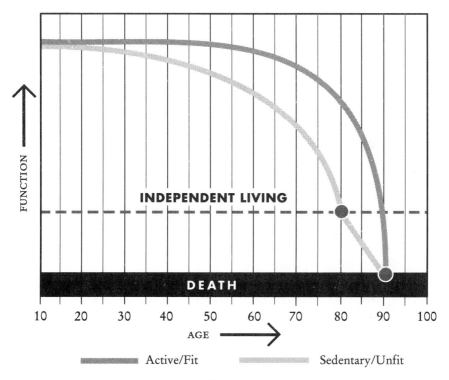

SOURCE: Institute for Aerobics Research, *The Strength Connection.*

WALKING AND YOUTH

If lifelong physical-fitness habits were taught at the beginning of life's spectrum, fewer people would be victims of compressed morbidity and loss of functional mobility at the end of it. Physical education as taught in schools is supposed to educate young people to understand and practice lifelong physical fitness. On close inspection, however, it appears that the effort is falling short in many respects.

Way back on May 16, 1986, *USA Today*, in a story headed "Help Kids Get Fit; Their Health Matters," reported, "Only about a third of students have a daily PE class." Segueing to September 13, 1990, in another story on youth fitness, *USA Today* reported that a survey showed that not much had improved. For most PE students, in-class time is too cluttered with administrative duties, specific skill instruction, and waiting in line. One study showed that "the students are physically active only about 27% of the time they're in PE." On balance, not only is physical education not reaching enough young people but even those who are taking it are not getting much activity.

In both *USA Today* stories, physical-fitness experts were quoted about what an appropriate PE class is. In the 1990 story, Dr. Lyle Micheli, president of the American College of Sports Medicine, put it bluntly: "Sports fitness is very different from health fitness. . . . Sports fitness is largely congenitally determined and contributes nothing to lifelong good health." Dr. Micheli is correct. Too much emphasis in high schools is placed on team sports, which involve only 5 percent; the other 95 percent of the student population is left standing on the sidelines. In an effort to get this group physically active, some schools are trying to develop "innovative, inclusive programs." As an example, one Arizona PE instructor said, "We do aerobics to music, jump ropes, go through obstacle courses, and climb ropes."

In *USA Today*'s 1986 youth-fitness story, a physical education expert said, "Instead of concentrating only on team sports, school PE programs should emphasize aerobics and activities that promote lifelong physical fitness such as jogging, swimming, and tennis." A chairman of the exercise-science department of a major southeastern university told *USA Today* that "quality PE programs should prepare kids to be physically active adults. . . . My preference would be specific skills that lead to lifetime fitness." The common thread of these recommendations is that children should be learning something they can and will do for a lifetime.

What is it that adults should do for a lifetime of fitness? As the statistics from *Healthy People 2000* revealed in Chapter 1, most adults don't do much of anything—and the older they get the less they do. Of those adults who do exercise, however, the largest number nationally are *walkers*. There are over three times as many walkers as joggers and runners. The number of adults who skip ropes and climb ropes for the long term is probably too small to be statistically significant. But if walking is the prevalent exercise for adults, why is it omitted from school PE programs?

In the fall of 1988, I found out. I conducted aerobic-walking classes for the sophomores, juniors, and seniors at St. Joseph's three high schools. None of their PE teachers knew anything about high-intensity walking, nor did the students. The whole thought of walking fast was foreign to them. In addition, the *attitudes* of high school students today are vastly different than they were when I went to high school in the 1940s. Eagerness to learn seems to be largely absent. Several English and math teachers confirmed this when I asked them about it. The results of my efforts at these grade levels were disappointing.

In the fall of 1989, I made another attempt to teach aerobic walking in the St. Joseph schools, but this time at the fifth-, sixth-, and seventh-grade levels. What a difference! These young minds were still inquisitive about life and eager to try new challenges. We had such fun that I believe it is a grievous omission not to make aerobic walking a fundamental part of PE for the early grades. If it is properly instituted there, it can ultimately be integrated into high school programs as children progress to that level.

In about 15 or 20 minutes, I taught the kids correct posture and the bent-arm-swing technique. Most of them were loose and rhythmic and picked it up quickly. Even several boys and girls bordering on obesity moved with good posture and rhythm. Those children will never be runners or rope jumpers, but, with proper coaching and encouragement, they could learn aerobic walking, an exercise that would help them control their weight problems for the rest of their lives. Aerobic walking is exactly what the 10-year-old in Chapter 12 needed. Where better to learn a lifetime exercise than in school?

After the youngsters became familiar with the bent-arm-swing technique, I lined the boys and girls in separate columns. The PE teacher stood 40 yards away and a boy and girl race-walked to the finish line. Most of the contests were close, and in the sixth grade of one school more girls won than boys. The kids had a good time and cheered for their sex to win.

Backing up my experience, in its November–December 1990

issue, *The Walking Magazine* reported on a pilot walking program in New York City. The Metropolitan Athletics Congress for the first time included race walking as a track and field event for elementary and junior high grades, open to students 8 to 13 years old at twenty-one schools in lower Manhattan. The kids trained for an 800-meter race before going on to a series of competitions that culminated in district championships, where Olympic-style medals were awarded. Although it was called race walking, I doubt that they learned the total technique as described in Chapter 9; nevertheless, the kids loved it. One 12-year-old girl was a four-time winner in the 800-meter event. She said, "The program helped me discover a talent I never knew I had. . . . At first, a lot of us thought race walking wasn't as important as the other track and field events, but now I think it's even harder since you have to concentrate so much on form." The program director of the Metropolitan Athletics Congress said, "Next to the 100-meter run, the race walk has become the most popular track and field event. . . . The kids love it." Over 400 youngsters were involved in the event.

Whether we call it race walking or aerobic walking, the kids have their arms bent and are walking as fast as they can. Unlike with running, they are not going to injure themselves; more important, they are learning an exercise that they can and should do for a lifetime.

Perhaps my cynicism at age 64 is showing through, but as this chapter is being written in the summer of 1991, many states and cities, along with the federal government, are facing huge budget deficits. Teachers are being laid off and school programs cut. One of the first classes to be cut is physical education. If all the kids are going to learn are things like rope jumping, so what? It costs nothing extra, however, to take a recess hour and have kids walk for 30 minutes. It doesn't take a Ph.D. in exercise physiology to teach aerobic walking. If approached, I believe many organized walking clubs would send volunteers to teach it at schools in their area.

In October and November of 1988, *The Physician and Sportsmedicine* ran a two-part series on the state of unfitness and childhood obesity in this country. In the articles, a National Children and Youth Fitness Study revealed that "American children today have more body fat than their counterparts twenty years ago. . . . Virtually all children (97.0%) are enrolled in physical education classes, but only 36.4% take those classes daily." In addition, the study reported, "The less time schools allow for physical education, the more time they allow for recess. . . . This suggests that schools are using recess as a substitute for physical education." If this is the case, children are getting shortchanged on an important part of their education.

The increase in body fat overall in children, and specifically the increase in childhood obesity, is a national problem that needs to be addressed. *The Physician and Sportsmedicine* stated: "Childhood obesity can cause emotional problems, elevate blood pressure, and—most importantly—lead to adult obesity, which is extremely difficult to reverse." Fat parents have fat children—who become fat parents. It is an unhealthy, sometimes deadly cycle. The subject of obesity is too complex to discuss in detail here, except to say that one of the main ways of controlling obesity is adequate, sustainable exercise.

Exclusion of moderate- to high-intensity walking from PE programs indicates that school officials and exercise professionals still can't fully comprehend how fundamental and effective exercise walking is. From fifth-graders to 80-year-olds—and for all ages in between—exercise walking truly is the one and only lifetime exercise.

15

THE
COMPLETE
EXERCISE

It is not commonly known, but the walking gait can work its magic from the neck up as well as from the neck down. The least publicized application of exercise is the role that it plays in the management of mental stress and anxiety. All too often exercise is emphasized only for weight control and cardiovascular fitness. The right kind of exercise, however, will relieve tensions, elevate self-esteem, dissipate hostilities, and build self-confidence. I say "right kind" because I have tried them all, but only walking works for me. Being on an exercise cycle, for instance, heightened my frustrations and made me count the minutes until I could quit. Walking, by contrast, is a natural tranquilizer.

If you experience stress or anxiety, take your troubled mind for a walk. A long walk is nature's catharsis for the emotional strains that creep into our lives. A daily walk is the anesthesia for life's pain and the antidote for life's poisons. Walking, preferably outside, will let you cut the mechanical and electrical umbilical cords of the machines and screens that connect you to the modern world. It will take you back, physically and mentally, to life's natural pace. The intensity of your walk will automatically match your level of stress. Anger, for instance, will succumb to a fast pace. I have never started a walk angry and ended up with the same feeling that I had when I began. You can literally walk your anger into the ground.

In our sedentary life-style, the human body, both physically and mentally, is starved for exercise or for some form of regular physical activity. The Greek physician Hippocrates, who is called the father of medicine, said, "All parts of the body which have a function, if used in moderation and exercised in labours in which each is accustomed, become thereby healthy, well developed and age more slowly, but if unused and left idle, they become liable to disease, defective in growth and age quickly." Hippocrates made that observation about 2,400 years ago. His words are even more relevant today.

As you contemplate the role of exercise in your life, heed the words of Hippocrates. He said that all parts of the body that have a function should be "exercised in labours in which each is accustomed." Walking fits his description perfectly. In the animal kingdom, your upright walking gait makes you unique. You are biomechanically engineered to be a walker. No exercise machine or arbitrarily designed physical-fitness routine can duplicate the all-encompassing beneficial effects that a good walk will contribute to your total well-being. Your body is its own perfectly balanced, self-contained exercise machine. It only needs you to put it in motion.

Anything further I might say at this point about the many health benefits of exercise walking would be redundant. If I don't have you convinced by now, another 100,000 words won't do so. There is one aspect of exercise walking that does need repeating, however, only because it is so difficult to get people to believe it: it makes you feel good. Without exception, all the exercise walkers I know say that they sleep better at night and have a higher energy level during the day, greater self-confidence, a more positive outlook on life, better mental acuity—*and they feel good!*

I mentioned at the beginning of this book that a daily walk is the best medicine of all for the body, mind, and spirit. As a walker, you will find that it is nearly impossible to walk daily in the outdoors without engaging in spiritual introspection. If, as I am, you are able to walk in rural areas and observe the beauty of nature, you will find that the mind tends to seek a higher meaning to existence than this brief journey we call life. You may find, as I have, that in addition to its physical and mental benefits, a daily walk can also be a time of spiritual fulfillment. For me it is prayer time and time to commune with my Creator as I walk under the big, beautiful dome of His outdoor cathedral.

To make a final point, I have searched in vain for something other than the overused cliché "can't see the forest for the trees." Unfortunately, that, better than any other choice of words, describes so many people's ongoing quest for an exercise or exercise machine that is better than walking. Starting with a slow 30-minute-per-mile stroll, and going down to the race-walking world record for the mile (5 minutes, 33.5 seconds), better than any other exercise the walking gait provides an unparalleled range of injury-free exercise and athletic challenge. In the forest of exercises and exercise machines, walking is the tallest tree of all; it is the only *complete exercise*.

We must part now, but I hope this book will motivate you to start walking for your body, mind, and spirit. Perhaps our paths will cross again someday and we can share a walk together. In the meantime, good health to you always.

A SELECTED BIBLIOGRAPHY

Alexander, R. McNeill. "Elastic Mechanisms in the Locomotion of Vertebrates." *Netherlands Journal of Zoology,* 1990.

———. "Human Walking and Running." *Journal of Biological Education,* 1984.

———. "Walking and Running." *American Scientist,* July–Aug. 1984.

Alexander, R. McNeill, R. F. Ker, M. B. Bennett, S. R. Bibby, and R. C. Kester. "Foot Strike and the Properties of the Human Heel Pad." *Journal of Engineering in Medicine,* Pt. H, 1989.

———. "The Spring in the Arch of the Human Foot." *Nature,* Jan. 1987.

Alexander, R. McNeill, and Alexandra Vernon. "The Dimensions of Knee and Ankle Muscles and the Forces They Exert." *Journal of Human Movement Studies,* 1975.

Alter, Michael J. *Sports Stretch.* Champaign, IL: Leisure Press, 1990.

American College of Sports Medicine. *Guidelines for Exercise Testing and Prescription,* 4th ed. Philadelphia: Lea & Febiger, 1991.

American Physical Therapy Association. "The Secret of Good Posture." Mar. 1991.

American Running and Fitness Association, Paul M. Taylor, and Diane K. Taylor. *Conquering Athletic Injuries.* Champaign, IL: Leisure Press, 1988.

Blair, Steven N. *Living with Exercise.* Dallas: American Health Publishing, 1991.

Bowman, Bob. *U.S. Race Walking Handbook 1991.* Indianapolis: The Athletic Congress/USA, 1991.

Cavagna, G. A., and R. Margaria. "Mechanics of Walking." *Journal of Applied Physiology,* 1966.

"Complete Injury Prevention Program at Last." *Runner's World*, Feb. 1991.

Cooper, Kenneth H. *The Aerobics Program for Total Well-being*. New York: Bantam, 1983.

"Do Ape-Size Legs Mean Ape-like Gait?" *Science*, 5 Aug. 1983.

Evans, William, and Irwin H. Rosenberg. "Boosting Your Biomarkers of Youth." *Prevention*, Mar. 1991.

Fixx, James. *The Complete Book of Running*. New York: Random House, 1977.

Gordon, Neil F. *Arthritis: Exercising Your Options*. Champaign, IL: Human Kinetics, in press.

———. *Diabetes: Exercising Your Options*. Champaign, IL: Human Kinetics, in press.

Gordon, Neil F., and Larry W. Gibbons. *The Cooper Clinic Cardiac Rehabilitation Program*. New York: Simon & Schuster, 1990.

Gould, Stephen Jay. "Enigmas of the Small Shellies." *Natural History*, Oct. 1990.

Henderson, Joe. *Jog, Run, Race*. Mountainview, CA: World Publications, 1977.

Inman, Verne T., Henry J. Ralston, and Frank Todd. *Human Walking*. Baltimore: Williams & Wilkins, 1981.

Johanson, Donald C., and Edey Maitland. *Lucy: The Beginnings of Humankind*. New York: Simon & Schuster, 1981.

Lovejoy, C. Owen. "Evolution of Human Walking." *Scientific American*, Nov. 1988.

———. "The Origin of Man." *Science*, 23 Jan. 1981.

Lovejoy, C. Owen, G. Heiple Kingsbury, and Albert H. Burnstein. "The Gait of Australopithecus." *American Journal of Physical Anthropology*, July 1973.

Lovejoy, C. Owen, and Rogert G. Tague. "The Obstetric Pelvis of A.L. 288-1 (Lucy)." *Journal of Human Evolution*, May 1986.

McArdle, William D., Frank I. Katch, and Victor L. Katch. *Exercise Physiology: Energy, Nutrition, and Human Performance*, 2nd ed. Philadelphia: Lea & Febiger, 1986.

Margaria, A. *Biomechanics and Energetics of Muscular Exercise.* Oxford: Clarendon Press, 1976.

Menier, D. R., and L. G. C. E. Pugh. "The Relation of Oxygen Intake and Velocity of Walking and Running in Competition Walkers." *Journal of Physiology* (London), 1968.

Meyers, Casey. *Aerobic Walking.* New York: Random House, 1987.

"Physical Fitness and All-Cause Mortality: A Prospective Study of Healthy Men and Women." *Journal of the American Medical Association*, 3 Nov. 1989.

Physician and Sportsmedicine, The, editors and contributors. "The Benefits of Walking." Sept. 1986.

———. "Characteristics of National-Class Race Walkers." Sept. 1981.

———. "Exercise Can't Always Counteract Your Diet." May 1990.

———. "Exercise Medicine in Medical Education in the United States." Oct. 1988.

———. "Exercise Roundtable." May 1985.

———. "Flexibility for the Knees." Feb. 1990.

———. "Flexibility for the Middle and Low Back." Oct. 1989.

———. "Getting Fit for Life: Can Exercise Reduce Stress?" June 1988.

———. "How I Manage Shin Splints." Dec. 1990.

———. "How Much Should I Exercise?" July 1989.

———. "Keeping Pace with the Many Forms of Walking." Aug. 1988.

———. "President Bush: He's Busy but He Still Makes Time for Exercise." July 1990.

———. "So, You Hate to Run . . ." Mar. 1990.

———. "Sports Medicine: Where Do We Go from Here?" June 1988.

———. "Strength and Endurance of the Lower Leg Muscles." Aug. 1989.

———. "Training Habits and Injury Experience in Distance Runners: Age-and-Sex-Related Factors." June 1988.

———. "Upper Body Exercise: 'Jarming' Instead of Jogging." May 1986.

Public Health Reports—Journal of the U.S. Public Health Service. "Special Section: Public Health Aspects of Physical Activity and Exercise." Mar.–Apr. 1985.

Rippe, James, Ann Ward, John Porcari, Patty Freedson, Stephanie O'Hanley, and Sharon Wilkie. "The Cardiovascular Benefits of Walking." *Practical Cardiology,* Jan. 1989.

Rooney, James R. *Biomechanics of Lameness in Horses.* Baltimore: Williams & Wilkins, 1969.

Rudow, Martin. *Advanced Race Walking.* Seattle: Technique Publications, 1987.

Running & FitNews [American Running and Fitness Association].

———. "Running Injuries During Infantry Training." Vol. 8, no. 11.

———. "Running Style." Vol. 9, no. 2.

———. "Warm-ups and Stretches Don't Prevent Muscle Soreness." Vol. 8, no. 7.

"Search for Early Man, The." *National Geographic,* Nov. 1985.

Sheehan, George. "The Best Advice for 400 Years." *Runner's World,* June 1987.

———. "Health vs. Fitness." *The Runner.* June 1987.

———. *Personal Best.* Emmaus, PA: Rodale Press, 1989.

———. "Walking: Underrated Training Aid." *The Physician and Sportsmedicine,* Sept. 1990.

"Slow Healing Fractures." *Runner's World.* Nov. 1986.

Solomon, Henry A. *The Exercise Myth.* New York: Harcourt Brace Jovanovich, 1984.

Strength Connection, The. Institute for Aerobics Research, 1990.

"To Live Longer, Take a Walk." *Newsweek,* 13 Nov. 1989.

University of California at Berkeley Wellness Letter, editors. "All of Us Are Athletes . . ." May 1991.

U.S. Department of Health and Human Services. *Healthy People 2000: National Health Promotion and Disease Prevention Objectives.* 1990.

Wagman, Richard J., and the J. G. Ferguson editorial staff. *The Medical and Health Encyclopedia.* Chicago: J. G. Ferguson, 1987.

"Walking for Exercise and Pleasure." President's Council on Physical Fitness and Sports, undated booklet.

Weil, Lowell S. "Aches and Pains of Running." Undated booklet.

INDEX

About the Author

CASEY MEYERS is a retired businessman who found a second career as a health-and-fitness writer after the publication in 1987 of *Aerobic Walking*, his first book. Since then he has conducted over 150 lectures and walking clinics for more than seven thousand people throughout the United States, including regular monthly walking clinics for the Cooper Wellness Program at Dr. Kenneth Cooper's Aerobics Center in Dallas, Texas. Mr. Meyers is also the walking consultant for NaturalSport walking shoes, and lives in St. Joseph, Missouri.